Oxford AQA GCSE History

Health and the People

c1000–Present Day

AUTHORS

J. A. Cloake

Aaron Wilkes

SERIES EDITOR

Aaron Wilkes

CONSULTANT

J. A. Cloake

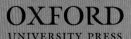

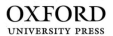

OXFORD
UNIVERSITY PRESS

Great Clarendon Street, Oxford, OX2 6DP, United Kingdom

Oxford University Press is a department of the University of Oxford.

It furthers the University's objective of excellence in research, scholarship, and education by publishing worldwide. Oxford is a registered trade mark of Oxford University Press in the UK and in certain other countries.

British Library Cataloguing in Publication Data

Data available

978-138-202310-8

Digital edition 978-138-202311-5

1 3 5 7 9 10 8 6 4 2

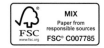

Paper used in the production of this book is a natural, recyclable product made from wood grown in sustainable forests.

The manufacturing process conforms to the environmental regulations of the country of origin.

Printed in Great Britain by Bell and Bain Ltd, Glasgow

Acknowledgements

The publisher would like to thank Jon Cloake for his work on the first edition of the Student Book on which this second edition is based. The publisher would also like to thank Chris Edge, Ben Fuller (Holocaust Educational Trust) and David Rawlings for their contribution in the development of this book.

The publishers would like to thank the following for permissions to use their photographs:

Cover: Daily Mirror/Mirrorpix/Mirrorpix via Getty Images.
Photos: p6(tl): Wellcome Collection. Attribution 4.0 International (CC BY 4.0); **p6(tr):** Guildhall Library & Art Gallery/Heritage Images/ Getty Images; **p6(bl):** Pictures from History / Bridgeman Images; **p6(br):** Photo 12 / Alamy Stock Photo; **p7(tl):** The Granger Collection / Alamy Stock Photo; **p7(tr):** Pictorial Press Ltd / Alamy Stock Photo; **p7(ml):** Otto Herschan Collection / Stringer/Getty Images; **p7(mr):** ZEPHYR/Science Photo Library; **p8:** Pictures from History / Bridgeman Images; **p9:** Archives Charmet / Bridgeman Images; **p10:** Everett Collection Historical / Alamy Stock Photo; **p11:** World History Archive / Alamy Stock Photo; **p13(tl):** Wellcome Collection. Attribution 4.0 International (CC BY 4.0); **p13(ml):** CPA Media Pte Ltd / Alamy Stock Photo; **p13(tr):** Art Directors & TRIP / Alamy Stock Photo; **p13(bl):** Bridgeman Images; **p14:** Album / Alamy Stock Photo; **p15:** Bibliotheque Nationale, Paris, France / Archives Charmet / Bridgeman Images; **p16:** Look and Learn / Bridgeman Images; **p19:** Robert Thom/American Pharmacists Association Foundation; **p21:** The Picture Art Collection / Alamy Stock Photo; **p22:** Photo 12 / Alamy Stock Photo; **p24(bl):**

Approval message from AQA

This textbook has been approved by AQA for use with our qualification. This means that we have checked that it broadly covers the specification and we are satisfied with the overall quality. Full details of our approval process can be found on our website.

We approve textbooks because we know how important it is for teachers and students to have the right resources to support their teaching and learning. However, the publisher is ultimately responsible for the editorial control and quality of this book.

Please note that when teaching the AQA GCSE History course, you must refer to AQA's specification as your definitive source of information. While this book has been written to match the specification, it cannot provide complete coverage of every aspect of the course.

A wide range of other useful resources can be found on the relevant subject pages of our website: www.aqa.org.uk.

Buyenlarge/Getty Images; **p24(mr):** Apic/Getty Images; **p25:** Heritage Image Partnership Ltd / Alamy Stock Photo; **p26:** Robert Thom / Alamy Stock Photo; **p27:** Wellcome Collection. Attribution 4.0 International (CC BY 4.0); **p28:** Robert Thom / Alamy Stock Photo; **p29(l):** Chronicle / Alamy Stock Photo; **p29(r):** Wellcome Collection. Attribution 4.0 International (CC BY 4.0); **p30:** PRISMA ARCHIVO / Alamy Stock Photo; **p31(l):** Wellcome Collection. Attribution 4.0 International (CC BY 4.0); **p31(r):** Library of Congress Prints and Photographs Division Washington, D.C. 20540 USA ; **p32:** Rijksmuseum/Bequest of L. Dupper Wzn., Dordrecht; **p33:** Wellcome Collection. Public domain.; **p34:** World History Archive / Alamy Stock Photo; **p35(t):** Bettmann/Getty Images; **p35(b):** Heritage Image Partnership Ltd / Alamy Stock Photo; **p36:** Guildhall Library & Art Gallery/Heritage Images/Getty Images; **p37:** Pictorial Press Ltd / Alamy Stock Photo; **p38:** Science History Images / Alamy Stock Photo; **p40:** Wellcome Collection. Attribution 4.0 International (CC BY 4.0); **p42:** Peter Horree / Alamy Stock Photo; **p43:** World History Archive / Alamy Stock Photo; **p45:** Everett Collection Historical / Alamy Stock Photo; **p46:** Chronicle / Alamy Stock Photo; **p47:** Amoret Tanner / Alamy Stock Photo; **p48:** Wellcome Collection. Attribution 4.0 International (CC BY 4.0); **p49:** Chronicle / Alamy Stock Photo; **p50:** The Granger Collection / Alamy Stock Photo; **p52:** Hulton Archive/Getty Images; **p53:** BSIP SA / Alamy Stock Photo; **p54:** Chronicle / Alamy Stock Photo; **p56:** Pictorial Press Ltd / Alamy Stock Photo; **p57(m):** Chronicle / Alamy Stock Photo; **p59(t):** Antiqua Print Gallery / Alamy Stock Photo; **p59(b):** Granger Historical Picture Archive / Alamy Stock Photo; **p60:** Science History Images / Alamy Stock Photo; **p61:** Otto Herschan Collection / Stringer/Getty Images; **p63:** Pictorial Press Ltd / Alamy Stock Photo; **p64:** Bettmann/CORBIS/ Bettmann Archive/Getty Images; **p65:** Bettmann/Getty Images; **p67(l):** Indiapicture / Alamy Stock Photo; **p67(r):** ZEPHYR/Science Photo Library; **p68:** Jeremy Sutton-Hibbert / Alamy Stock Photo; **p69:** Science & Society Picture Library/Getty Images; **p71:** Christopher Pillitz/Alamy Stock Photo; **p74(l):** Trinity Mirror / Mirrorpix / Alamy Stock Photo; **p74(r):** LH Images / Alamy Stock Photo; **p77:** The National Archives; **p78:** Heritage Image Partnership Ltd / Alamy Stock Photo; **p81:** Pictorial Press Ltd / Alamy Stock Photo; **p86:** World History Archive / Alamy Stock Photo; **p92:** Punch Cartoon Library / TopFoto.

Artwork by Q2A Media Services Pvt. Ltd.

We are grateful to the authors and publishers for use of extracts from their titles and in particular to the following:

AQA for practice questions from the AQA GCSE History Paper 2 'Shaping the Nation', copyright © 2015 AQA and its licensors. AQA accepts no responsibility for the study tips given which have neither been provided nor approved by AQA.

We have made every effort to trace and contact all copyright holders before publication, but if notified of any errors or omissions, the publisher will be happy to rectify these at the earliest opportunity.

Links to third party websites are provided by Oxford in good faith and for information only. Oxford disclaims any responsibility for the materials contained in any third party website referenced in this work.

Contents

Health and the People c1000–Present Day

Introduction to the Oxford AQA GCSE History series

The Oxford AQA GCSE History series has been specially written by an expert team of teachers and historians with examining experience to match each part of your AQA course. The chapters which follow are laid out according to the content of the AQA specification. Written in an interesting and engaging style, each of the eye-catching double-pages is clearly organised to provide you with a logical route through the historical content.

There is a lively mix of visual **Sources** and **Interpretations** to enhance and challenge your learning and understanding of the history. Extensive use of photographs, diagrams, cartoons, charts and maps allows you to practise using a variety of sources as evidence.

The **Work** activities and **Practice Questions** have been written to help you check your understanding of the content, develop your skills as a historian, and help you prepare not just for GCSE examinations, but for any future studies. You can develop your knowledge and practise examination skills further through the interactive activities, history skills animations, practice questions, revision checklists and more on *Kerboodle**.

Britain: Health and the People c1000–Present Day

This book guides you through one of AQA's Thematic Studies, Britain: Health and the People c1000–Present Day. Thematic studies focus on key developments in the history of Britain over a long period of time. You will look at the importance of factors such as war, superstition and religion, government, communication, science and technology and the role of the individual, and how these factors impact upon society.

Understanding history requires not just knowledge, but also a good grasp of concepts such as causation, consequence and change. This book is designed to help you think historically, and features primary sources; these sources will help you think about how historians base their understanding on the careful evaluation of evidence from the past.

We hope you'll enjoy your study of Health and the People –

Jon Cloake
Series Consultant

Aaron Wilkes
Series Editor

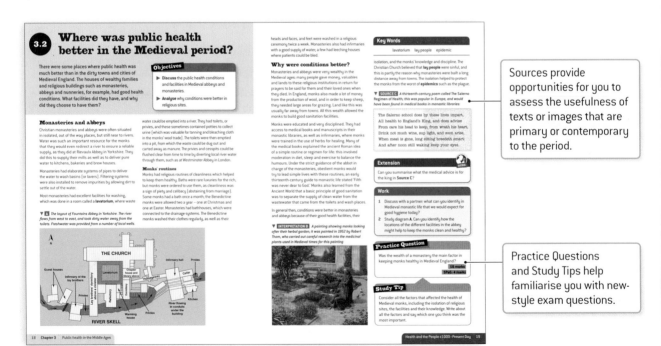

Sources provide opportunities for you to assess the usefulness of texts or images that are primary or contemporary to the period.

Practice Questions and Study Tips help familiarise you with new-style exam questions.

*Kerboodle is not approved by AQA.

How to use this book

Written for the new AQA specification, the features in this book include:

Objectives

At the beginning of the sections, you will find a list of learning objectives. These are based on the requirements of the course.

▼ SOURCE ▼ INTERPRETATION

Sources introduce you to material that is primary or contemporary to the period, and **Interpretations** provide you with various people's different perspectives on the past.

Practice Question

These are focused questions to help you practise your history skills, including evaluating sources and essay writing. They give you an idea of the types of questions you might get in an examination.

Study Tip

These are hints to highlight key parts of **Practice Questions** and will help you answer the questions.

Fact

Fascinating references, facts or anecdotes that will make you think and add to your knowledge and understanding.

Work

The activities and questions aim to develop your knowledge, understanding and key history skills. They are designed to be progressive in terms of difficulty, and to get you to think about the topic, become familiar with the history, and apply what you have learned.

Extension

This is an opportunity to challenge you to investigate the history more deeply through independent research and reflection.

Key Words

The important phrases and terms are highlighted and are also defined in the glossary. Learn what they mean – and how to spell and use them correctly.

Timeline

A short list of dates identifying key events to help you understand chronological developments.

Key Biography

Details of a key person to help you understand the individuals who have helped shape history.

Timeline

Britain: Health and the People

This thematic study covers over 1000 years in the history of medicine and public health in Britain. You will explore how medicine and public health changed, why change happened when it did, whether change brought progress, and the significance of the changes. You will also consider how factors — such as war, chance, religion, science and technology — sometimes worked together to bring about particular developments at a particular time; and what their impact upon society was. And although the focus of this study is the development of medicine and public health in Britain, it will draw on wider world ideas and events to show how they affected medicine and public health in Britain over this long sweep of history.

Fact

Historians sometimes add a 'c' before dates. This stands for 'circa', which means 'around' or 'approximately'.

c1230
Compendium Medicine is written by Gilbert Eagle – a comprehensive English medical textbook blending European and Arab knowledge of medicine

1628
William Harvey proves the circulation of the blood

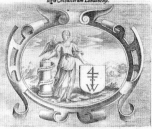

1724
Guy's Hospital is founded in London

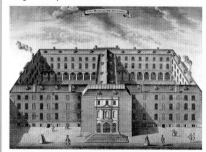

1600

1700

1300

1200

1250
This illustration shows a Medieval doctor checking the patient's urine and pulse

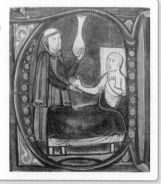

1348
Black Death arrives in England

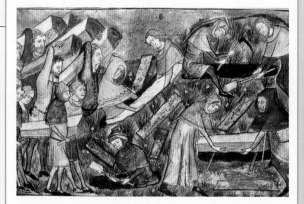

1882
Robert Koch's work on the identification of tuberculosis is publicised in Britain

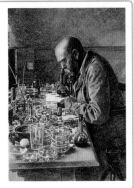

1928
Alexander Fleming discovers that penicillin kills bacteria

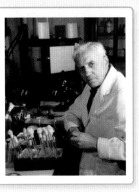

1978
First 'test-tube' baby is born

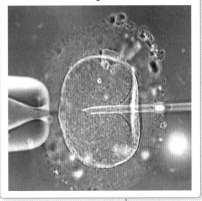

1858
Joseph Bazalgette begins building a network of sewers under London's streets

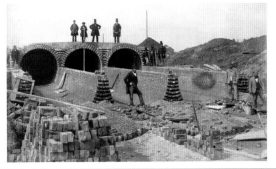

1847
James Simpson uses chloroform as an anaesthetic

1848
First Public Health Act is introduced

1953
Francis Crick and James Watson publish their research on the structure of DNA

2000

1900

1800

1963
First liver transplant is carried out in America

1798
Edward Jenner develops cowpox as a protection against smallpox

1867
Joseph Lister publishes a description of carbolic antiseptic in surgery

1948
NHS comes into operation

1951
Rosalind Franklin captures the pattern of DNA in a photograph

2003
Human Genome Project is declared complete with the final sequencing of the entire human genome; this is a huge breakthrough in understanding how genes help determine who a person is

1906
First of the Liberal social reforms – including free school meals for the poorest children, free medical checks and free treatment – is introduced

2019
An outbreak of COVID-19 (a contagious respiratory disease) is identified in China. It is recognised as a pandemic (an infectious disease that spreads across the world) by the World Health Organisation (WHO) in March 2020.

1.1 What did a Medieval doctor know?

This book focuses on the development of medicine and public health in Britain from Medieval times (also known as the Middle Ages, c1000–1500), to the present day. Of course, even before the Medieval period in Europe, people had tried to cure illness in the **Ancient World**. The ideas of famous Greek doctors like Hippocrates and Galen had been passed on and became an essential part of the treatments used by a Medieval doctor. To understand this history, and the importance of medical ideas from the Ancient World, you will need to understand where Medieval people went for medical advice.

Objectives

▶ **Outline** what a Medieval doctor knew, including natural, supernatural, Hippocratic and Galenic ideas.

▶ **Explain** what training Medieval doctors received.

▶ **Examine** the medical options for a poor or rich person in the Medieval period.

Fact

The Medieval period, AD500–1500, can be divided into the Early Middle Ages, the High Middle Ages and the Late Middle Ages. This book starts in the High Middle Ages. Medical ideas from the Ancient World were lost in the Early Middle Ages because of wars, but by the High Middle Ages Europe had become more peaceful and stable, so medical knowledge found its way back into Europe from the Islamic world.

If you were ill in Medieval England, there were many people to go to for treatment. It was a medical marketplace, from the local wise woman to the **barber-surgeon** in the town, and – if you could afford it – a university-trained doctor.

What could a Medieval doctor do?

Medieval doctors followed the ancient Greek method of 'clinical observation', or bedside observation of the patient, to produce a **diagnosis** of the disease. By the Medieval period, rather than noting all the symptoms, doctors tended to concentrate on just two indicators: they only took the pulse and noted the colour, smell, and taste of the urine. From this, the doctor might prescribe natural medicines made from plants, animal products, spices, oils, wines, and rocks.

A common treatment was **bloodletting** (or 'purging'), which was when blood was removed by opening a vein or using **leeches** to suck it out. The cure didn't often work, because the blood had to be taken from exactly the right spot on the body. Other treatments might involve giving you something to make you vomit or go to the toilet. Remedies often combined natural with supernatural approaches, such as prayers, charms and **astrology**.

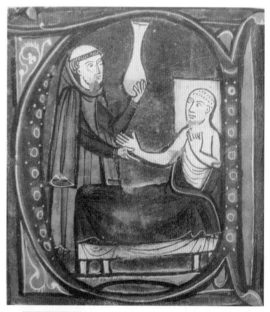

▲ **SOURCE A** *An illustration from a book published in 1250 showing a Medieval doctor examining a patient's urine and checking his pulse*

The four humours: beliefs about the cause of illness

Medieval doctors based their natural cures on the ancient Greek theory of illness, which involved the equal balance of four '**humours**' within the body. They believed that a person became ill when the humours were out of balance, and the doctor's job was to restore this balance. If there was too much blood, then the patient would be bled; if there was not enough they might be advised to drink more red wine. The theory of the four humours fitted what the Medieval doctor could observe.

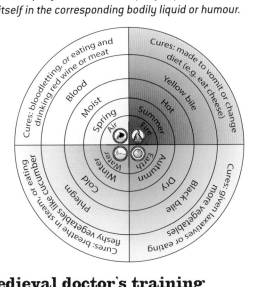

▼ **B** *According to the theory of the four humours, each element was strongest in a specific season, with specific qualities. The element showed itself in the corresponding bodily liquid or humour.*

A Medieval doctor's training

To qualify as a doctor in the Middle Ages could take at least seven years of study at a university like Oxford or Cambridge. The doctors learned mainly by listening to lectures and debating what they had read about in books. It was possible for a fully qualified doctor to leave university without having seen an actual patient.

Doctors in Britain learned the treatments of Hippocrates and Galen, together with the medical knowledge from the Muslim, Indian and Chinese worlds. They studied British medical textbooks, such as Gilbert Eagle's *Compendium Medicine* (c1230), which were based on Greek knowledge: they dealt with each part of the body working from the head downwards, and brought together medical theory, recipes, charms and Christian prayers.

Who did ordinary people turn to?

There were few university-trained doctors in Medieval England, and they were expensive. Less respected but more common were the barber-surgeons in towns. For most people who lived in small villages there would be a wise woman or man who offered traditional remedies for illness. The wise people used a mixture of natural herbal remedies, first aid and supernatural cures. Their knowledge would be passed down by word-of-mouth, but some was written down. One of the earliest remedy books was the Anglo-Saxon manuscript *Leech Book of Bald* (950). In markets and fairs there would be many people offering herbal potions; some would pull teeth, mend dislocated limbs or perhaps even set a fracture in splints.

Christianity was very central to Medieval people's lives, so sick people might also turn to the local monastery or the parish priest for medical help. People at the time believed that God could send illness as a punishment for wickedness and crimes, so prayers and charms were often used as remedies. Prayers were often made to Christian saints who were said to cure specific ailments.

Key Words

Ancient World   barber-surgeon   diagnosis
bloodletting   leech   astrology   humours

▼ **SOURCE C** *An illustration from 1450, showing a treatment using the four humours theory*

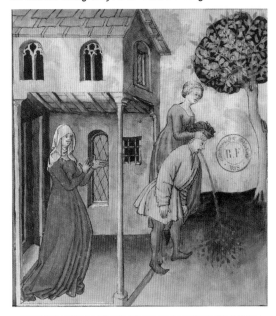

Work

1   Where could you find medical advice in the Medieval period if you were a) poor or b) rich?

2   Where did a Medieval doctor's knowledge come from?

3   List at least two ways in which medical knowledge was passed on in the Medieval period.

4   Study **Source C**. What do you think this treatment is trying to cure?

5   In your own words, explain how a patient could be treated using the theory of the four humours.

6   Discuss with a partner: what are the obvious differences between Medieval doctors and modern doctors today?

Extension

Research some of the Medieval saints that people prayed to in order to make them better or to protect them from illness. You could start with Saint Lucy, Saint Anthony or Saint John of Bridlington.

2.1 How did Christianity affect Medieval medicine?

Throughout the Medieval period, Christianity was the only main religion in Western Europe. The Christian Church was a powerful organisation that influenced the decisions of kings and emperors, and possessed great wealth. It advised both ordinary and great people about how they should live their lives. What were Christian attitudes towards the sick? And did the Church help or hinder medical progress in the Medieval period?

Objectives

▶ **Outline** Christian ideas about medicine.

▶ **Explain** how the sick were treated by the Christian Church, including the role of hospitals.

▶ **Assess** the contribution of Christianity to medical progress in Medieval Britain.

What were Christian ideas about health and medicine?

The Christian Church believed in following the example of Jesus, who healed the sick. For this reason, Christians believed that it was good to look after the sick, and so they founded many hospitals. However, there was a strong belief that illnesses came from God, and curing an illness would be a challenge to God who had sent it as a punishment or a test of faith. So, it was important to care for the patient, not necessarily cure them.

Prayers to God were therefore the most important treatment: 'To buy drugs or to consult with physicians doesn't fit with religion,' said Saint Bernard, a famous twelfth-century Christian monk. The Church also encouraged the belief in miraculous healing. There were many shrines filled with relics of the bones, hair and other body parts of a holy person. These shrines were places that people made **pilgrimage** to, for help with their illnesses, such as the shrine of Saint Thomas Becket at Canterbury.

While the Church valued prayers, it also respected the traditional medical knowledge of the Ancient World because it thought Hippocratic and Galenic ideas were correct. Monks preserved and studied these ideas: they copied out the books by hand, as well as traditional medical books like Pliny's *Natural History*, which was an encyclopaedia of everyday family remedies.

How did Christians treat the sick?

Between 1000 and 1500, more than 700 hospitals were started in England. Many hospitals were centres of rest where sick people might recover in quiet and clean surroundings. Some were small, with enough space for only 12 patients (the same number as Jesus had disciples). Many hospitals did not have doctors but a chaplain (a priest), and were run by monks or nuns to a strict pattern of diet and prayer.

Hospitals depended on charity for money, and were mainly financed by the Christian Church or by a wealthy **patron**. There were several different types of hospitals: for example, there were hospitals or asylums for the mentally ill, such as Bedlam in London. Monasteries had infirmaries (small dormitory wards) that could provide free treatment to the sick and the poor. There were a few large hospitals, such as St Leonard's in York.

▼ **SOURCE A** An illustration, from c1500, of the Hotel Dieu in Paris, a late Medieval hospital; the French king's doctors worked there

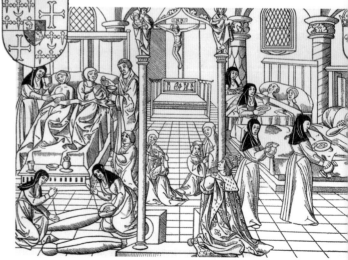

Key Words

pilgrimage   patron   leprosy   contagious   crusading order

Fact

St Leonard's Hospital was built during the reign of the Norman King Stephen (1135–54). By 1370, St Leonard's could look after over 200 sick people. From the time of the Normans, the hospital enjoyed the patronage of kings and the right to collect special taxes from the surrounding area.

There were also special hospitals called 'Lazar houses' that dealt with people who had **leprosy**. The disease was **contagious**, so to prevent people catching it, leprosy hospitals were set up outside towns. In England these 'houses' were often started by the **crusading orders** such as the Knights Templar in the twelfth century, because many crusaders caught the disease, which was widespread in the Middle East at the time.

Did Christianity help or hinder medical progress in the Medieval period?

In Europe, the training of doctors began after 1200, when the continent became more peaceful and prosperous. The Christian Church controlled the universities because that was where religion was studied and where Church leaders were trained; medicine was usually the second subject studied after religion. In Britain, the Church controlled the training of doctors in the universities of Oxford and Cambridge. There they taught the medical ideas of the ancient Greeks and Romans. The training was to make the old knowledge clear and understandable; it was not to discover new ideas.

The Christian Church approved of Galen's books because he believed in a single god: this fitted with Christian ideas (although Galen himself did not identify as a Christian). However this meant that it was difficult to challenge anything that Galen wrote, as it would be seen as a criticism of the Church. Church attitudes to new ideas were shown by what happened to the thirteenth-century English monk, Roger Bacon. He was arrested for his ideas. He suggested that original scientific experimentation was important.

Ultimately, the Church saw the role of the doctor not as a healer, but as someone who could predict the symptoms and duration of an illness, and provide the reasons for why God might inflict the illness on the person. This gave people comfort, and allowed patients and their families to put their affairs in order and die in peace. As Faritius, the famous eleventh-century doctor and abbot of Abingdon, said to the family of a little boy who died under his care, 'there is no medicine for death.'

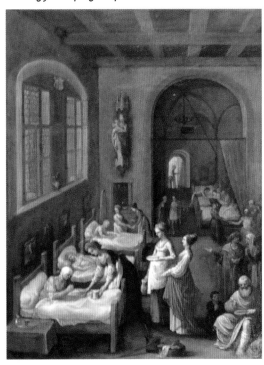

▼ **SOURCE B** *A sixteenth-century painting showing Saint Elizabeth of Hungary (tending to the patient, bottom left), who was famous in the thirteenth century for helping the poor and the sick*

Work

1   What did Medieval Christians think caused illnesses?

2   How did Christians treat sick people in Medieval times? Try to identify three points.

3   Study **Source A**. Describe what you can see in the hospital. How does it support what you have read about Medieval hospitals?

4   Do you agree or disagree that the Christian Church held back medical progress? Explain your answer.

Practice Question

How useful is **Source B** for understanding Christian ideas about illness?   **8 marks**

Study Tip

In a 'how useful' type of question about a visual source, remember to consider what the provenance tells you as well as what you can learn from the image.

How did Islam affect Medieval medicine?

Western Europe entered a period known as the Early Medieval period when the Roman Empire lost its power. At this time, Islam became the main religion in the Middle East and North Africa. Led by its Prophet, Muhammad, the followers of Islam established an enormous and unified Islamic Empire. During the height of Islam's culture and learning from c750–1050, Islamic doctors made great contributions to medical knowledge. What did they contribute to medical science? And why were they able to do so?

▼ **A** *A map showing the extent of the Islamic Empire by 750*

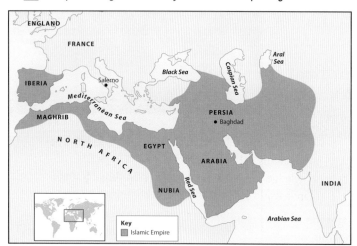

The Islamic Empire was a single state ruled by one man, known as the **Caliph**. Caliphs provided the peace and order needed for medical progress. Moreover, many Caliphs were interested in science and supported Islamic medicine. During the reign of Caliph Harun al-Rashid (786–809), the capital city of Baghdad became a centre for the translation of Greek manuscripts into the language of Islam: Arabic. The Caliph's library preserved hundreds of ancient Greek medical books by Hippocrates and Galen, which were lost to Western Europe during the Early Middle Ages. Al-Rashid's son, Caliph al-Mamun (813–33), developed his father's library into 'The House of Wisdom', which was the world's largest library at the time, and a study centre for scholars. The Islamic religion itself encouraged medical learning: Prophet Muhammad inspired people to 'seek learning even as far as China' and said, 'For every disease, Allah has given a cure.' So, scientists were encouraged to discover those cures.

What were Islamic ideas on health and medicine?

In the Islamic Empire the first hospitals were set up for people with mental illnesses. These people were treated with compassion as victims of an unfortunate illness. This was very different from how Christian doctors thought of them – as being punished by God.

In 805, Caliph al-Rashid set up a major new hospital in Baghdad with a medical school and a library. Unlike Medieval Christian hospitals, this was intended to treat the patients, and not simply care for them. Hospitals called bimaristans were built in many Islamic cities to provide medical care for everyone: men and women, rich and poor, Muslim and non-Muslim. Doctors were permanently present and medical students trained alongside them.

Did Islam help or hinder medical progress in the Medieval period?

Two Muslim doctors in particular, Rhazes and Avicenna, had a great influence on medicine in Western Europe. Their discoveries, along with the old medical knowledge of the ancient Greeks, first found their way to Western Europe in the Middle Ages. This was through the Latin translations of a merchant named Constantine the African, who arrived in Italy around 1065. Gerard of Cremona, an Italian translator, continued this work in the twelfth century with the first Latin translation of Avicenna's book, *Canon of Medicine*. The universities in Padua and Bologna in Italy soon became the best places to study medicine in Europe. These medical ideas reached England through trade, as merchants brought new equipment, drugs and books.

Al-Razi (c865–c925)

Known in Western Europe as Rhazes, he stressed the need for careful observation of the patient, and distinguished measles from smallpox for the first time. He wrote over 150 books. Although a follower of Galen, he thought that all students should improve on the work of their teacher. One of his books was called *Doubts about Galen*.

Ibn al-Nafis (1213–1288)

Born in Damascus, Syria, this Muslim physician is considered to be the first to describe how blood circulated around the body via the lungs. Galen thought that blood passed straight from the right-hand side of the heart to the left-hand side, but Ibn al-Nafis concluded that Galen was wrong. He wrote about many medical topics (including eye diseases and diet) but his books were not read in the West – and Europeans continued to accept Galen's mistake until the seventeenth century. To find out more about the move away from Galen's ideas, read pages 30–31.

Ibn Sina (980–1037)

Also known as Avicenna, he wrote a great encyclopaedia of medicine known as *Canon of Medicine*. Comprising over a million words, it covered the whole of ancient Greek and Islamic medical knowledge at the time. It listed the medical properties of 760 different drugs, and contained chapters on medical problems such as anorexia and obesity. It became the standard European medical textbook used to teach doctors in the West until the seventeenth century.

The influence of Islamic medicine

Key Words

Caliph

▼ **SOURCE B** *From the front cover of a fourteenth-century Italian copy of Avicenna's* Canon of Medicine

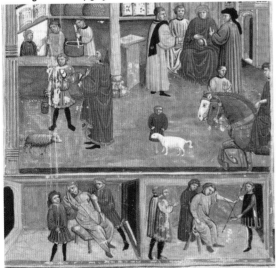

Extension

As well as preserving the writings of the ancient Greeks and Romans, Islamic doctors added their own, new knowledge. Research some of the new drugs from the Islamic world such as camphor, laudanum, naphtha and senna.

Work

1   Identify three things that Islam believed about medicine and illness.

2   Study the provenance of **Source B** and what is happening in the picture. How does it link to what you have learned?

3   Did Islam help or hinder medical progress? Explain your answer using the following factors: government, ideas, science, communication, individuals.

Practice Question

Was the preservation of the writings of the ancient Greeks and Romans the most important contribution that Islam made to medical progress?   **16 marks**
SPaG: 4 marks

Study Tip

What do you think were the different contributions that Islam made to medical progress? You might consider the scientific approach, the new drugs, the books, the discoveries, or the hospitals. Write about several contributions and then explain which one you think was the most important.

How good was Medieval surgery?

Surgery in the Medieval period was a risky business. Surgeons had no idea that dirt carried disease. Some believed it was good to cause pus in wounds, and operations were done without effective painkillers. Surgery was limited, since surgeons could not help patients with deep wounds to the body: these patients would die from bleeding, shock and infection. What kind of surgery occurred then? Did any surgeons make progress during the Medieval period?

Objectives

▶ **Describe** who did surgery in Western Europe and the Islamic Empire during the Medieval period.

▶ **Explain** what types of surgery could be done at the time.

▶ **Evaluate** the medical progress achieved in surgery.

Who practised surgery?

Many Medieval surgeons were not surgeons in the modern sense. Most were barbers who combined hair cutting with small surgical operations such as bloodletting and tooth extraction. Compared with doctors, barber-surgeons were lower class medical tradesmen. Surgeons learned their skill by being apprenticed to another surgeon, watching and copying them; or they learned on the battlefield since wars were frequent in the Medieval period.

What could a Medieval surgeon do?

The most common surgical procedure was bloodletting, which was done to restore the balance of humours in the body. It was performed by making a small cut on the inside of the arm, from which the blood was allowed to run out. Amputation, or the cutting off of a painful or damaged part of the body, was another common treatment. It was known to be successful in cases of breast cancer, bladder stones, and haemorrhoids. In Medieval times, it was thought that epilepsy was caused by demons inside the brain – so a surgeon might cure an epileptic patient by drilling a hole into the skull to let the demon out!

SOURCE A *A fourteenth-century illustration of* **trepanning**

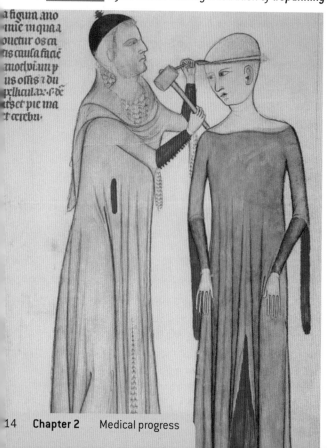

Most surgery took place on battlefields. In everyday life, surgery was performed as a last resort. Patients faced the problem of pain and shock in operations. Some attempts were made to put the patient to sleep, but more often than not the patient had to be held or tied down. Surgeons used natural substances such as mandrake root, opium and hemlock as **anaesthetics** for their operations, but too strong a dose might kill the patient. **Cauterisation** was a very common method of burning the wound to stop the flow of blood: it was usually done with a heated iron and was immensely painful. A surgeon would have many different tools: saws for amputation, arrow pullers, cautery irons and bloodletting knives.

Who made progress in surgery during the Medieval period?

The science of surgery in Western Europe and in the Islamic Empire was advanced during the Medieval period by surgical pioneers who tried new methods. Their books were read in Latin by educated and religious men in Europe; in England, they were translated into English. By the end of the fourteenth century, English doctors and surgeons could read about the ideas of many surgeons. Some examples follow.

Abulcasis

Abulcasis, a Muslim surgeon considered the 'father of modern surgery', wrote a 30-volume medical book, *Al Tasrif*, in 1000. He invented 26 new surgical instruments and described many new procedures, including using ligatures for tying off blood vessels. He made cauterisation popular.

A fifteenth-century illustration of the surgeon Abulcasis and his assistant cauterising a mouth wound

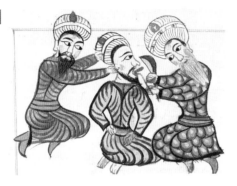

Frugardi

Roger Frugardi of Salerno, Italy, wrote a textbook on surgery called *The Practice of Surgery* in 1180. It was widely used in Europe. Frugardi warned against trepanning, tried ambitious operations on the chest, and attempted to remove bladder stones.

Hugh of Lucca and his son Theodoric

Hugh of Lucca and his son Theodoric were famous surgeons who worked at Bologna University, Italy. They wrote a book in 1267 criticising the common view that pus was needed for a wound to heal. They used wine on wounds to reduce the chances of infection and had new methods of removing arrows. Despite being ahead of their time, their ideas about preventing infection went against Hippocratic advice and did not become popular.

Mondino

There was a new interest in **anatomy** in the fourteenth century. In 1315, a public **dissection** was allowed in Bologna, supervised by Mondino de Luzzi, a famous professor. In 1316, Mondino wrote the book *Anathomia*, which became the standard dissection manual for over 200 years. Dissections were introduced in most European universities to train doctors and to show them that Galen was correct. Even if the body did not fit Galen's description, they did not doubt Galen: people believed that the body must be wrong!

De Chauliac

One of the most famous surgeons of the Medieval period was the French surgeon, Guy De Chauliac. His famous textbook *Great Surgery* (1363) dominated English and French surgical knowledge for 200 years. The textbook contains references to Greek and Islamic writers like Avicenna; he quoted Galen about 890 times. He did not like Theodoric of Lucca's ideas about preventing infection and he wrote about his opinion in detail in his book, which was the main reason that Lucca's ideas did not catch on.

John of Arderne

John of Arderne was the most famous surgeon in Medieval England. His surgical manual, *Practica* (1376), contained illustrations of his operations and instruments. It was based on Greek and Arab knowledge and his experience in the Hundred Years War between England and France. He used opium and henbane to dull pain. He charged a large fee for an operation he developed to treat an anal abscess (swelling with pus), a condition common in knights who spent long periods on horseback. In 1368, he tried to separate the surgeons from lower-class barbers by forming a work association called The Guild of Surgeons within the City of London.

Work

1 a Who carried out most surgery in the Medieval period?
   b How did they learn their trade?
2 What were the two most common surgical procedures?
3 Three problems for the surgeon are to take away pain, prevent infection and stop bleeding. Discuss in pairs or in groups: what were the traditional solutions of most Medieval surgeons to these three surgical problems?

Extension

Do you think there was any progress in surgery during the Medieval period? Explain your answer.

Where was public health worse in the Medieval period?

Public health refers to the health and well being of the population as a whole, in a particular place and at a particular time. People often assume that conditions in Medieval towns were awful. They were certainly poor by modern standards, but the levels of cleanliness and hygiene were rising in some places during the Medieval period. How were these improvements made? Why were there problems with public health? To what extent did people care about cleanliness?

Objectives

▶ **Describe** the public health conditions in Medieval towns.

▶ **Explain** attitudes to public health in Medieval England.

▶ **Assess** the quality of public health in Medieval towns.

What was public health like?

Medieval towns were built near rivers or other bodies of water, because they needed easy access to water; rivers also provided a means of transport. There were various systems of water supply in Medieval towns. Most people got their water from local springs, wells or rivers. Some towns had elaborate systems built by the Romans to supply water, which still worked well. However, as towns grew, the existing systems could not cope with the increased demand for water. So, Medieval towns such as Exeter and London used new technology with pipes made of wood or lead.

Many town dwellers also used rivers and streams to remove their sewage and other waste. Sometimes, however, people just threw their toilet waste onto the street, along with other household rubbish.

Most towns and some private houses had **privies** (a toilet located in a small shed outside a house or building), with **cesspits** underneath where the sewage was collected. In some towns, people left money in their wills so that public privies for the town's citizens could be built and maintained. Cesspits would be dug out annually by **gong farmers**, and like dung heaps, they were a valuable source of manure. If they were not emptied regularly, the sewage from these cesspits easily seeped into and polluted rivers and wells.

Towns were generally dirty places. There were some paved streets, but in small towns, streets became muddy when it rained. In addition, the open drains that ran down street centres to carry away water and waste would often overflow. In a downpour, privy cesspits might also overflow, leaving excrement spread over the road. Streets outside the houses of wealthier citizens were swept by their servants and were therefore cleaner, but in poorer areas the streets stank and were often littered with waste.

Keeping towns clean

Between 1250 and 1530, the number of towns in England grew as the population rose, which put pressure on public health facilities. Mayors and councillors knew that improvements would be expensive, but they did not want to become unpopular by increasing local taxes to fund these improvements.

▼ **INTERPRETATION A** *A Medieval street scene, drawn by an artist in 1962*

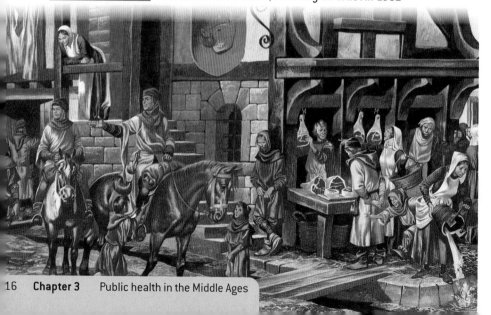

Also, the lack of sanitation was partly because people had no knowledge of germs and their link to disease and infection. They did think, however, that disease was spread by 'bad air', so they were keen to remove unpleasant smells.

Rivers provided water to businesses such as bakeries and breweries, which also used the rivers to remove their waste. Town councils tried to stop businesses from polluting rivers in this way, but this was difficult. In towns, people lived side-by-side with businesses. Leather tanners, for example, used dangerous chemicals and smelled awful, while meat butchers created waste products such as blood and guts, which were then dumped into rivers. Local craft guilds tried to restrict the skilled workers' activities to certain areas, and to regulate the nuisances that their tradesmen caused. In Worcester, for example, a law of 1466 said that the entrails and blood of butchered animals had to be carried away that same night.

What did town councils do?

Some Medieval town councils in England tried to keep the environment clean and healthy. They passed various local laws encouraging people to keep the streets in front of their houses clean and to remove their rubbish, but it was not easy to maintain cleanliness.

▼ **SOURCE B** *From the records of a London Court case in 1321:*

> The jury decided that Ebbegate Lane used to be a public passage. Master Thomas Wytte and William de Hockele built privies projecting out from the walls of their houses. From the privies human filth falls onto the heads of the passers-by and blocks the passageway.

Key Words

public health   privy   cesspit   gong farmer

Work

1 What were the most important sources of water in a Medieval town?
2 a Identify three things in Medieval towns that were a threat to people's health.
   b Identify three things in Medieval towns that might have kept people healthy.
3 Study **Interpretation A**. What can you see in it that you have learned about from these two pages?
4 Read **Source B** carefully. What offence has been committed here?

Practice Question

Explain two ways in which public health in a Medieval town and public health in a Medieval monastery were different.   **8 marks**

Study Tip

In your answer refer to the water supply, dealing with sewage, and attitudes to cleanliness in each place.

Timeline

1298	1330	1371	1374	1388
King Edward I complains that unhygienic conditions in York are a danger to his soldiers preparing for invasion, so the council orders the building of public latrines in the city	Glamorgan council passes laws to stop butchers throwing animal remains into the High Street, and orders that no one should throw waste onto the streets or close to the town gates	The London mayors and councillors try to make the city healthier by prohibiting the killing of large animals within the city walls	The London local council gives up trying to control building and sewage disposal over the Walbrook stream. Instead they make householders who use the stream pay a fee to have it cleaned each year	Parliament passes a law which fines people £20 for throwing 'dung garbage and entrails' into ditches, ponds, and rivers. However, it is not easy to make people obey the laws nor to catch those who disobey them

Where was public health better in the Medieval period?

There were some places where public health was much better than in the dirty towns and cities of Medieval England. The houses of wealthy families and religious buildings such as monasteries, abbeys and nunneries, for example, had good health conditions. What facilities did they have, and why did they choose to have them?

Objectives

▶ **Discuss** the public health conditions and facilities in Medieval abbeys and monasteries.

▶ **Analyse** why conditions were better in religious sites.

Monasteries and abbeys

Christian monasteries and abbeys were often situated in isolated, out of the way places, but still near to rivers. Water was such an important resource for the monks that they would even redirect a river to ensure a reliable supply, as they did at Rievaulx Abbey in Yorkshire. They did this to supply their mills as well as to deliver pure water to kitchens, bakeries and brew houses.

Monasteries had elaborate systems of pipes to deliver the water to wash basins (or lavers). Filtering systems were also installed to remove impurities by allowing dirt to settle out of the water.

Most monasteries had excellent facilities for washing, which was done in a room called a **lavatorium**, where waste water could be emptied into a river. They had toilets, or privies, and these sometimes contained potties to collect urine (which was valuable for tanning and bleaching cloth in the monks' wool trade). The toilets were then emptied into a pit, from which the waste could be dug out and carted away as manure. The privies and cesspits could be flushed clear from time to time by diverting local river water through them, such as at Westminster Abbey in London.

Monks' routines

Monks had religious routines of cleanliness which helped to keep them healthy. Baths were rare luxuries for the rich, but monks were ordered to use them, as cleanliness was a sign of piety and celibacy (abstaining from marriage). Some monks had a bath once a month; the Benedictine monks were allowed two a year – one at Christmas and one at Easter. Monasteries had bathhouses, which were connected to the drainage systems. The Benedictine monks washed their clothes regularly, as well as their

▼ **A** *The layout of Fountains Abbey in Yorkshire. The river flows from west to east, and took dirty water away from the toilets. Freshwater was provided from a number of local wells.*

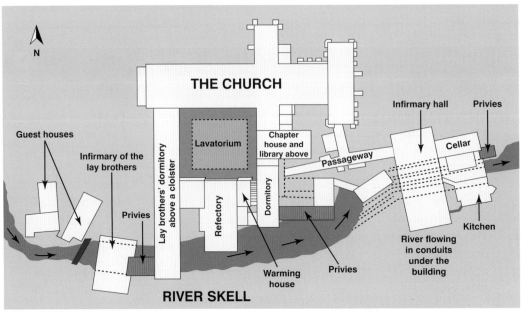

heads and faces, and feet were washed in a religious ceremony twice a week. Monasteries also had infirmaries with a good supply of water; a few had leeching houses where patients could be bled.

Why were conditions better?

Monasteries and abbeys were very wealthy in the Medieval ages: many people gave money, valuables and lands to these religious institutions in return for prayers to be said for them and their loved ones when they died. In England, monks also made a lot of money from the production of wool, and in order to keep sheep, they needed large areas for grazing. Land like this was usually far away from towns. All this wealth allowed the monks to build good sanitation facilities.

Monks were educated and very disciplined. They had access to medical books and manuscripts in their monastic libraries, as well as infirmaries, where monks were trained in the use of herbs for healing. Many of the medical books explained the ancient Roman idea of a simple routine or regimen for life: this involved moderation in diet, sleep and exercise to balance the humours. Under the strict guidance of the abbot in charge of the monasteries, obedient monks would try to lead simple lives with these routines; an early thirteenth-century guide to monastic life stated 'Filth was never dear to God.' Monks also learned from the Ancient World that a basic principle of good sanitation was to separate the supply of clean water from the wastewater that came from the toilets and wash places.

In general then, conditions were better in monasteries and abbeys because of their good health facilities, their

▼ **INTERPRETATION B** *A painting showing monks looking after their herbal garden; it was painted in 1952 by Robert Thom, who carried out careful research into the medicinal plants used in Medieval times for this painting*

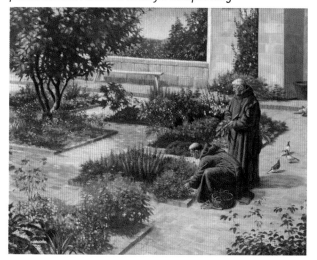

Key Words

lavatorium   lay people   epidemic

isolation, and the monks' knowledge and discipline. The Christian Church believed that **lay people** were sinful, and this is partly the reason why monasteries were built a long distance away from towns. The isolation helped to protect the monks from the worst of **epidemics** such as the plague.

▼ **SOURCE C** *A thirteenth-century poem called* The Salerno Regimen of Health; *this was popular in Europe, and would have been found in medical books in monastic libraries:*

> The Salerno school does by these lines impart,
> All health to England's King, and does advise
> From care his head to keep, from wrath his heart,
> Drink not much wine, sup light, and soon arise,
> When meat is gone, long sitting breedeth smart:
> And after noon still waking keep your eyes.

Extension

Can you summarise what the medical advice is for the king in **Source C**?

Work

1   Discuss with a partner: what can you identify in Medieval monastic life that we would expect for good hygiene today?

2   Study diagram **A**. Can you identify how the locations of the different facilities in the abbey might help to keep the monks clean and healthy?

Practice Question

Was the wealth of a monastery the main factor in keeping monks healthy in Medieval England?

16 marks

SPaG: 4 marks

Study Tip

Consider all the factors that affected the health of Medieval monks, including the isolation of religious sites, the facilities and their knowledge. Write about all the factors and say which one you think was the most important.

Consequences of poor public health: the Black Death

3.3A

The Black Death was an epidemic disease in the Medieval period; it began in Asia and travelled rapidly along the trade routes to Western Europe. It reached Constantinople (in modern day Turkey) in 1347 and arrived in England in 1348. The Black Death killed nearly half of Europe's population. In Britain, at least 1.5 million people died. What caused it, and why did it spread? Why were people so terrified of catching it?

Objectives

▶ **Describe** the main symptoms of the Black Death disease.

▶ **Explain** beliefs about its causes, treatment and prevention.

▶ **Evaluate** the impact of the disease.

The Black Death

Historians believe that the Black Death was a combination of both the **bubonic** and the **pneumonic plagues**. The bubonic plague was spread by fleas: buboes or lumps were found on a person's groin, neck and armpits. The lumps oozed pus and bled when opened, then a high fever and vomiting of blood would follow. The pneumonic plague was a more deadly form of disease: it infected the lungs, causing fever and coughing, and was spread by contact with a victim's breath or blood.

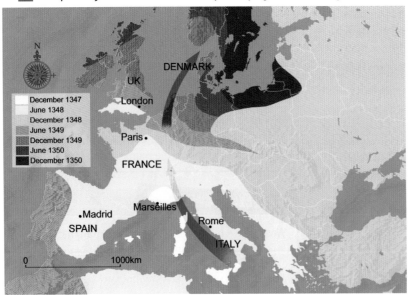

▼ **A** *The spread of Black Death across Europe; the plague reached England in 1348*

▼ **SOURCE B** *The Italian writer Boccaccio describes the symptoms of Black Death in 1348:*

The first signs of the plague were lumps in the groin or armpits. After this, livid black spots appeared on the arms and thighs and other parts of the body. Few recovered. Almost all died within three days, usually without any fever.

▼ **SOURCE C** *Robert of Avesbury, a chronicler at the Archbishop of Canterbury's court, wrote in 1349:*

The pestilence, which had first broken out in the land of the Saracens (the Middle East), became much stronger; it visited all the kingdoms with the scourge of sudden death. It began in England in Dorset, and immediately advancing from place to place attacked men without warning. Very many of those attacked in the morning were dead before noon. And no one it touched lived longer than three or four days. And reaching London, it deprived many of their life every day, and increased so greatly from February till April 1349 that there were more than 200 dead bodies a day buried in the new Smithfield cemetery. The grace of the Holy Spirit finally intervening, about May, 1349, it ceased in London.

What did people think caused the Black Death?

European doctors in the fourteenth century did not understand infections or how diseases were transmitted, so they could not explain the cause of the Black Death. They blamed it on the position of stars and planets, on bad air, and even on the poisoning of wells by Jews (none of these was true). Blaming the plague on Jews led to many attacks against Jewish communities in Europe, but this did not happen within England since, as a result of religious intolerance, King Edward I had expelled all the Jews in 1290. Many people were very religious, and they believed that God was punishing them for their sins: they thought that only God's anger could produce so many horrific deaths.

▼ **SOURCE D** *A fifteenth-century French painting showing Saint Sebastian praying on behalf of plague victims*

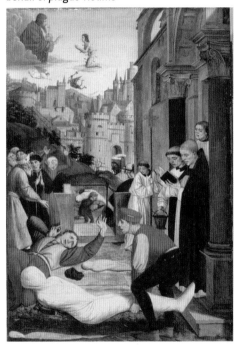

What really caused the Black Death?

The Black Death was thought to have been an outbreak of mainly bubonic plague caused by the **bacteria** *Yersinia pestis*. This bacteria thrived in the stomachs of fleas that lived on the blood of rats. When rats died of the plague, the fleas had to find a new host and moved on to humans. Death

could be very quick for weaker victims, such as those with malnutrition. In the Medieval period, food shortages were common, and the resulting high food prices meant people didn't eat well, which weakened people's immunity (their ability to fight infection).

The Black Death spread quickly due to several reasons: one was that in crowded ports and towns, people lived close together and knew nothing about contagious diseases. If the bubonic plague reached the lungs of the victim, then they could spread the pneumonic form of the plague to others, through the air, by coughing. The disposal of bodies was crude and helped to spread the disease still further, as those who handled the dead bodies did not protect themselves in any way. In villages, bodies that were hastily buried in shallow pits could be dug up by wild animals at night; the body parts would be spread around. The filth that littered streets gave rats the perfect environment to breed and increase in number.

Authorities had no idea what caused the plague. They had simple laws about keeping streets clean, but there was little enforcement of the laws, and few effective regular ways of cleaning the streets. People did not always practise cleanliness, and it was common to throw rubbish and human waste into the streets and rivers.

How did people try to deal with the plague?

No medical knowledge existed in Medieval England to cope with the disease. People tried anything to escape it, including drinking mercury, or shaving a chicken and strapping it to the buboes. Understandably, peasants were terrified at the news that the Black Death might be approaching their village or town. Some fled to other towns and villages. Most avoided contact with other people; local councils also tried to **quarantine** infected places.

Fact

One of the more extreme actions taken in Europe to prevent Black Death was flagellation: some people wanted to show their love of God by whipping themselves, hoping that God would forgive them their sins and that they would be spared. Flagellation was not welcomed in England.

Work

1 What was the main characteristic of the bubonic plague?
2 According to **Source C**, what made the Black Death a terrifying disease?
3 Identify two things that might have helped people avoid the plague, and two that would not.
4 What do you think is the reason why there were so many different incorrect explanations of the causes of Black Death at the time?

Consequences of poor public health: the Black Death

By the end of 1350, the Black Death had subsided, but it never really died out in England over the next few hundred years. There were further outbreaks in 1361–62, 1369, 1379–83, 1389–93, and throughout the first half of the fifteenth century. The plague is thought to have returned at intervals with varying degrees of deadliness until the eighteenth century. On its return in 1603, for example, the plague killed 38,000 Londoners, and it came again in the Great Plague of 1665. By the early nineteenth century, the threat of plague had diminished, but it was quickly replaced by a new disease – **cholera**.

The impact of the Black Death

The Black Death had a huge impact on society. In Medieval England, it killed at least a third of the population between 1348 and 1350. Older age groups were more easily affected, and experienced a higher number of deaths.

The Black Death had enormous economic and social consequences. Fields went unploughed as the peasants who usually did the farming became victims of the disease. Food was not harvested and it rotted in the fields; village farm animals were untended and escaped into forests. Whole villages were often wiped out by the plague, but those who survived often faced starvation.

Food shortages

Towns and cities too faced food shortages, as the nearby villages could not provide them with enough food. The Medieval lords (noble landowners) who lost their farmer peasants to the disease changed to sheep farming, since this required fewer workers. This change to sheep farming in turn reduced the supply of basic foods such as bread. As a result of the Black Death, inflation occurred: the price of food went up (because there was less of it around), creating more hardship for the poor. In some parts of England, food prices quadrupled, and became unaffordable.

Peasant wages

Laws at the time stated that peasants could only leave their village if they had their lord's permission. After the Black Death, many lords were desperately short of workers for their land, so they actively encouraged peasants to leave the village where they lived to come to work for them. When peasants did this, their new lord refused to return them to their original village. On the other hand, some of the peasants who survived the Black Death believed that God had specially protected them. Therefore, they took the opportunity to improve their lifestyle by demanding higher

▼ **SOURCE E** *Illustration in a fourteenth-century history book written by an abbot, recording the impact of the Black Death; it shows people carrying coffins*

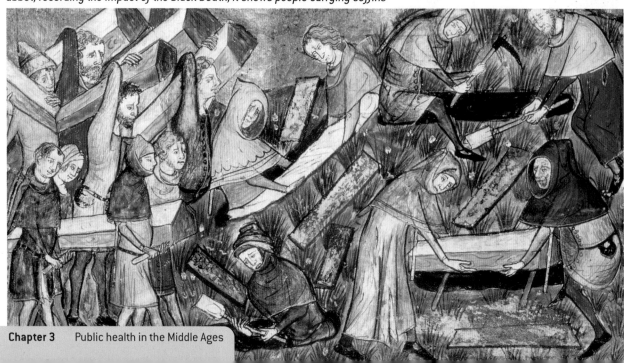

wages: they knew that lords were desperate to get their harvests in. All of this began to upset the idea of the **feudal system**, a form of Medieval land ownership that tied peasants to the land. So, an indirect consequence of the Black Death was that new laws were introduced, which caused anger and revolt among peasants. To curb peasants roaming around the countryside looking for better pay, the government introduced the Statute of Labourers in 1351.

▼ **SOURCE F** *Adapted from the Statute of Labourers, 1351:*

No peasants could be paid more than the wages paid in 1346. No lord or master should offer more wages than paid in 1346. No peasants could leave the village they belonged to.

Fact

Though some peasants ignored the Statute of Labourers, many knew that disobedience would lead to serious punishment. This created great anger, which was to boil over eventually in the Peasants' Revolt of 1381. A long-term cause of the revolt was that after the Black Death, the vastly reduced number of peasants found it harder to pay (and more bitterly resented) the new taxes that the king demanded to fund his wars abroad.

Another impact of the Black Death was that opinions about the Catholic Church changed: some of the churchmen were criticised for cowardice when they deserted their villages. However, this was balanced out by the vast number of priests who died. So, while the reputation of the Church was damaged, it also lost a great number of experienced clergy. It was a serious blow to the Catholic Church. Due to the misunderstanding of the causes of Black Death, there was also widespread persecution of minorities such as Jews, foreigners, beggars and lepers.

Fact

Can you catch the plague today?
From 1944–93, 362 cases of human plague were reported in the USA. The plague could become a major health threat again, but so far, only one case of drug-resistant plague has occurred (in Madagascar in 2014).

Key Words

cholera   feudal system

Work

1   When were there other outbreaks of plague in England?

2   In what ways did the plague affect the Catholic Church?

3   Create a mind-map showing the short-term and long-term consequences of the deaths of so many farmer peasants. You could also organise your consequences under headings, such as economic, social, cultural, and political.

4   'The number of people who died was the most important consequence of the Black Death.' Work with a partner to discuss this view. Do you agree with it? Why or why not? You could use your mind-map from Question 3 to help you answer this question.

Practice Question

How useful is **Source E** to a historian studying the impact of the Black Death in England?   **8 marks**

Study Tip

To answer this question, try to use the caption (provenance), and also describe what you can see is happening in the image.

Extension

In 2013, the tunnelling for London's new Crossrail station at Farringdon uncovered a plague pit belonging to the Charterhouse monastery. Scientists believe that so many bodies buried in such a short space of time must have meant the deaths were caused by pneumonic plague (with death rates of 90 to 100 per cent) rather than bubonic plague (with date rates of 50 per cent). Look up the research findings: in what ways did the discoveries add to or change historians' understanding of the Black Death and its impact?

4.1 What was the Renaissance?

Look carefully at Sources A and B. Source A is a drawing of the human body, from the Middle Ages. Source B is a drawing of the human body, made during the **Renaissance**. What are the differences between the two pictures? It seems obvious that the person who drew Source B knew more about the human body than the artist of Source A. Why was the artist able to create a more accurate picture? What has this to do with the Renaissance?

Objectives

▶ **Define** the term Renaissance.

▶ **Examine** the causes of the Renaissance.

▶ **Assess** the impact of the Renaissance on medicine.

Defining the Renaissance

The Renaissance is a term that describes a period in history that flourished in the late 1400s. It bridged the era between the Late Middle Ages and the Early Modern time, and began in Italy. At that time Italy was divided into a number of rich, powerful, independent city-states, one of which was Florence. In Florence, wealthy businessmen and traders were interested in the world of the ancient Greeks and Romans, and they paid educated scholars and artists to investigate it and translate it for them. The discoveries made by studying these ancient books both delighted and inspired the people who read them, but they also became critical of the many versions of the old texts. They wanted their knowledge to be based on an accurate, original version. This approach applied not only to old texts, but also to other aspects of their lives. People did not just accept what they were told, but began to ask questions, find evidence themselves and experiment with new ideas. Throughout Italy, people started to believe that being educated in art, music, science and literature could make life better for everyone. In fact, as people's interest in the ancient knowledge grew, many said the experience was a 'rebirth' of learning (the word 'renaissance' means 'rebirth' in Italian). The Renaissance changed the way people viewed their lives.

▼ **SOURCE B** Sketches of the human body, by Leonardo da Vinci; he was a Renaissance scientist, inventor, and painter who made over 30 human dissections

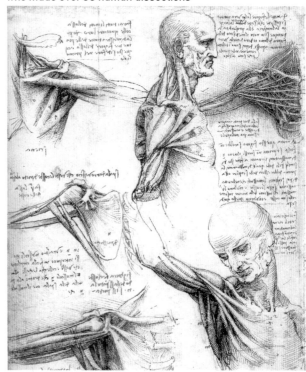

▼ **SOURCE A** A Medieval drawing of the human body

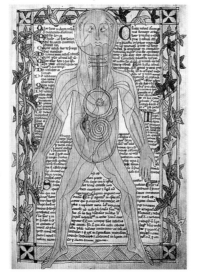

The Renaissance takes hold

The Renaissance was a cultural movement where people questioned accepted truths, searched for evidence, and experimented with new ideas. For centuries, people had accepted that the Church had all the answers to their questions. Now, many educated people wanted to find out for themselves and work out what the right answers were. Scientists experimented; traders explored new lands and made more accurate maps; doctors tried different treatments; and artists began using new methods to make their paintings more lifelike than ever.

How did the Renaissance spread?

Before the Renaissance, books were rare and expensive because they had to be copied out slowly by hand. This meant that knowledge was restricted to a few people who could afford or had access to books. As more people read about the Ancient World and experimented, they wanted to share their discoveries. A new invention made in 1451, the printing press, allowed them to do this: it printed pages far more quickly and accurately than before. As a result of the printing press, more people could read the ancient books as well as books about new discoveries.

Extension

One of the most difficult things historians have to do is to understand the way ideas affect events. Medicine is only one area of human knowledge you will learn about that was affected by the Renaissance. Find out how some other areas of knowledge, such as art, music, science or literature, developed because of the Renaissance. For example, you could look up the contributions of these Renaissance figures: Leonardo da Vinci, Thomas More, Erasmus or Copernicus.

Work

1 In your own words, state what was 'reborn' in the Renaissance.

2 How did the invention of the printing press affect the spread of Renaissance thinking?

3 How did Renaissance artists help progress in medicine?

4 Which of the consequences of the Renaissance would have the biggest impact on medical progress? Explain your answer.

Key Words

Renaissance

▼ **SOURCE C** *A printing press, c1500; the invention of the printing press can be compared to the invention of the Internet, as both allowed ideas and information to spread far more quickly than before*

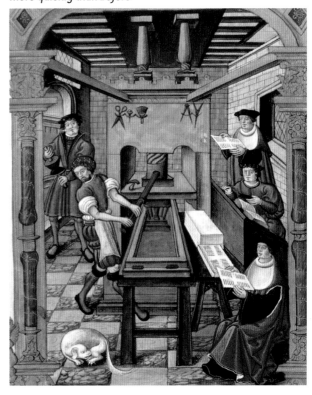

New inventions

New technology such as gunpowder meant injured soldiers got new types of wounds. As a result, doctors had to find new ways to deal with these wounds. Some used new scientific methods of learning to find out better ways to treat injuries.

New lands

Explorers, sailors and merchants used more accurate maps. The discovery of the Americas in the late 1400s showed the value of finding new things and making discoveries, rather than sticking to old ideas. New foods and medicines were also brought back from this 'new world'.

Consequences of the Renaissance

New learning

A scientific method of learning began, which involved observation, hypothesis and experimentation. Much of this started with doctors and scientists reading books from ancient Greece and Rome. Soon scholars began to question old established beliefs.

New ideas spread quickly

The printing press allowed new ideas to spread quickly around Europe, and old and new books to be studied.

New style of art

A new desire to show the human form in more realistic detail led artists to study the body more carefully.

4.2 The impact of the Renaissance on Britain: the work of Vesalius

In 1537, a young Belgian medical student called Andreas Vesalius published a book which completely supported the centuries-old views of the ancient Greek physician Galen about human anatomy. By 1543, the same student was a Professor of Anatomy, and published a revolutionary textbook which showed the many mistakes that Galen had made. What made Vesalius change his mind about Galen? The textbook transformed the teaching of anatomy. What was so revolutionary about his new book? How did Vesalius contribute to medical progress?

Andreas Vesalius (1514–64) was born in Belgium. His studies led him to the University of Paris, where he was taught by Jacob Sylvius, a professor who was a fanatical follower of Galen's teaching of anatomy (and who later became a fierce opponent of Vesalius' discoveries). Vesalius was a gifted student, and it was no surprise when he became Professor of Surgery at the University of Padua in Italy.

Unusually for the time, Vesalius did the dissections of the human body himself, rather than leaving it to an assistant. He carried out his own research to locate the best places for bloodletting. From his dissections, he began to realise that there were many mistakes in Galen's writing when compared with his own observations of the human body. For example, he saw there were no small holes in the heart.

Until this time, doctors had believed Galen had given a correct description of anatomy. Dissections had been carried out to prove Galen was right, not to check or challenge him. When other doctors observed the same differences that Vesalius noticed, they blamed either the particular body they were dissecting, or said that human anatomy had changed since Galen's times.

> ## Fact
>
> Galen (AD 131–201) was a famous Greek physician. His books showed important and often accurate observations on the human anatomy, including the heart, kidney and nerve functions. Galen's views dominated medical practice and how medicine was taught in universities for 1400 years.

▼ **INTERPRETATION A** *A 1962 painting, by Robert Thom, of Vesalius dissecting. He explains his observations, rather than simply reading Galen's descriptions aloud: his students found this a fascinating new way to learn.*

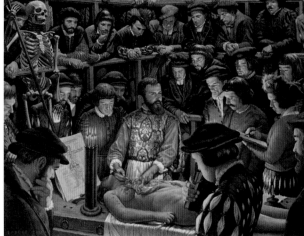

Vesalius and anatomy

Through careful observation, Vesalius realised that sometimes Galen's findings were wrong, because they were based on animal dissections rather than human ones. Vesalius also dissected animals to show how Galen had gained his knowledge: the breastbone in a human being has three parts, not seven as in an ape, for example. Vesalius' lectures were very popular. He promoted dissection as a way to discover more about the body, and as a way that students could learn about the body.

The knowledge that Vesalius gained from dissection was made available to everyone through his beautifully illustrated textbook *The Fabric of the Human Body* (1543). The illustrations were startlingly precise. Unlike previous anatomy books, which focussed on individual organs of the body, the textbook was organised differently to explain how the different systems within the body worked, such as the skeleton, the muscles, the nerves, the veins, digestion and reproduction. However, Vesalius faced heavy criticism for daring to say that Galen was wrong. He had to leave his job in Padua and later became a doctor for the Emperor Charles V.

Vesalius' contribution to medical progress in England

Vesalius' work soon found an appreciative audience in England. Within two years of publication, an Italian printer, Thomas Geminus, published *Compendiosa*, a book which copied all of Vesalius' illustrations. For the text, Geminus used the famous French surgeon, Henri de Mondeville's, 1312 book *Surgery*. Geminus sold his book to be used as a manual for barber-surgeons in London to learn their trade. *Compendiosa* was very popular in England, and three editions were published between 1545 and 1559. In the latter half of the sixteenth century, many copies of Vesalius' original book came to England, where they influenced and inspired English surgeons.

Vesalius' work overturned centuries of belief that Galen's study of anatomy was correct. He used the Renaissance approach because he based his work and writings on questioning and research on the human body itself. Through dissection and through his book, Vesalius shared new knowledge with the world. And although Vesalius' work did not lead to any medical cures, it was the basis for better treatments in the future. Vesalius showed others how to do proper dissections, and famous sixteenth-century anatomists who followed his approach, such as Fabricius, Realdo Columbo and Fallopius, used dissection to find out more about specific parts of the body.

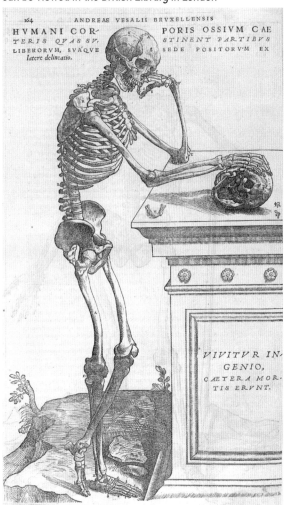

▼ **SOURCE B** *An illustration of the skeletal system in Vesalius' textbook; a copy of this rare and important work can be viewed in the British Library in London*

Fact

Henry VIII gave barber-surgeons a charter in 1540 to form the Company of Barber-Surgeons, making it a respectable and regulated profession. Through the charter, barber-surgeons were granted the corpses of four criminals every year for public dissection.

Work

1 What did Vesalius find out about Galen's work? Explain your answer carefully.

2 How does **Interpretation A** show what was new about Vesalius' approach to anatomy?

3 Why was Vesalius' textbook so revolutionary?

4 How did Vesalius have an immediate impact in England?

Practice Question

Explain two ways in which Medieval anatomy and Renaissance anatomy were different.

8 marks

Study Tip

Review what you have learned about Medieval anatomy from pages 14–15. You could refer to the knowledge they each had and the attitudes to dissection in both periods.

How important were Paré's discoveries?

In 1536, during the Battle of Milan, two injured soldiers were brought to the young French surgeon, Ambroise Paré. Their faces were disfigured and their clothes still smouldered from the gunpowder that had scorched them. Another soldier asked Paré if they could be helped. Sadly, Paré said they could not, because they were too badly wounded. The soldier went over to the wounded men and calmly slit their throats. Paré shouted at him but the soldier said, 'I pray that if I was ever in such a state someone would do the same for me so that I would not suffer as they did.'

Objectives

▶ **Consider** surgical knowledge before Paré and the challenge his work posed.

▶ **Describe** the methods and discoveries of Paré.

▶ **Examine** Paré's achievement and contribution to medical progress in England.

Ambroise Paré (1510–90) went on to be surgeon to four French kings, became the most famous surgeon in Europe, and published several books about his work. Paré had first learned surgery as an apprentice to his brother, who worked at a hospital in Paris. He then became a French army surgeon. How did Paré's experiences inspire him to make his discoveries?

Treating gunshot wounds and bleeding

In Paré's time, guns were fairly new inventions, so surgeons were not used to treating gunshot wounds. At first, surgeons thought gunshot wounds were poisonous, and the standard way of dealing with them was described in the influential book *Of Wounds in General* (1525) by Jean de Vigo. This stated that the wounds had to be burned out using boiling oil. On top of the pain of the wound, this treatment was agonising for the patient. Paré observed this and was upset by the suffering. During a French battle in 1537, when he ran out of hot oil, he improvised. Vigo recommended a cream of rose oil, egg white and turpentine be smeared over the wounds after cauterising with the burning oil. Without the oil, Paré used just the cream to soothe the patients. Despite his worries, Paré's patients slept well and their wounds healed quickly. Paré challenged accepted practice based on observation and experimentation, and wrote a book about treating wounds in new and better ways in 1545.

Another method Paré promoted was the use of ligatures (strings or threads) in amputations (cutting off a limb). The usual way of stopping bleeding was by cauterising a wound – putting a red-hot iron, called a cautery, on it.

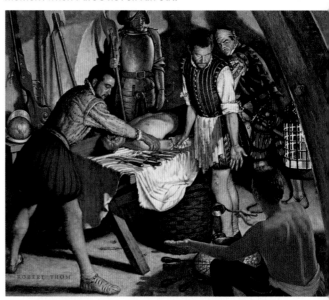

▼ **INTERPRETATION A** *Paré treating a wounded soldier, in a picture drawn in 1962 by Robert Thom. It shows the moment when Paré's hot oil ran out.*

Paré revived an old method to stop bleeding, by tying ligatures around individual blood vessels, recommended by Galen. This was very effective compared with cauterising, which he called the 'too cruel way of healing'. Paré also designed the *bec de corbin* or 'crow's beak clamp' to halt bleeding while the blood vessel was being tied off with a ligature. However, ligatures could introduce infection to a wound; they also took longer to implement than cauterising: speed was crucial during battle surgery. Due to the number of amputations that Paré had to do, he quickly moved on to designing and making false limbs for wounded soldiers, and included drawings of them in his writings.

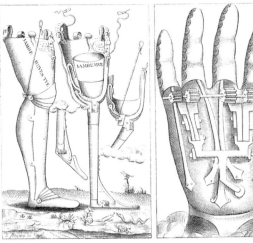

Fig. 1. — Jambes artificielles du temps d'Ambroise Paré.
(D'après une ancienne gravure.)

Fig. 2. — Main artificielle du temps d'Ambroise Paré.
(D'après une ancienne gravure.)

What was Paré's contribution to medical progress in England?

Paré admired, read and learned from the work of Andreas Vesalius. In his 1561 book *Anatomie Universelle* and his famous *Works on Surgery* (1575), Paré included large sections of Vesalius' work on anatomy. By translating Vesalius' writings from the original Latin into French, Paré greatly increased surgeons' understanding of anatomy, since most surgeons were not taught Latin. Paré's books soon circulated throughout Europe.

Paré's *Works on Surgery* was widely read by English surgeons in the original French, and an English hand-written translation of the book was given to the library of the Barber-Surgeons of London in 1591. This was long before it was printed in English in 1634.

In sixteenth-century England, there were a number of surgeons who followed Paré's Renaissance approach to surgery: these surgeons observed, questioned and experimented with new ideas. The most famous was William Clowes (1544–1604), surgeon to Queen Elizabeth I. He greatly admired Paré as the 'famous surgeon master', and like Paré, gained most of his medical experience on the battlefield. He was talented at stopping bleeding from wounds, and carried a vast number of healing potions in his medicine chest. He agreed with Paré that gunshot wounds were not poisonous. In 1588, he published his book *Proved Practice*, which shared his own knowledge about how to deal with battlefield wounds, especially those caused by gunpowder. Clowes also acknowledged Paré as the source for his treatments of burns using onions in 1596.

▼ SOURCE C *A picture from William Clowes' book,* Proved Practice, *showing the many chemical potions, mixtures and lotions in his medicine chest. He advised the Elizabethan navy surgeons on what to carry in their surgical chests, and is also credited with inventing a new paste that stopped the bleeding of wounds.*

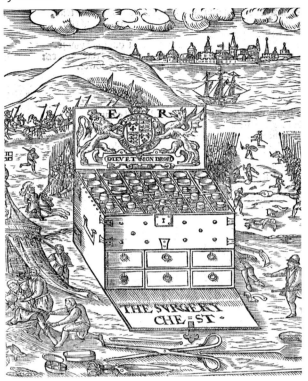

THE SVRGERY CHE=ST

Work

1 Describe in your own words the moment that the artist has captured in **Interpretation A**. What point do you think the artist is making?

2 Consider the statement: 'Paré was compassionate, resourceful, and skilled.'

   a How might his work show this?

   b Do you agree with the statement?

3 The spirit of the Renaissance was to do with observation, questioning and experimentation. In what ways did Paré's work show this?

4 Explain how each of the following factors contributed to the progress of medicine: chance; war; individual brilliance; technology; communication.

5 What was the impact of Paré's work in England?

6 Study **Source C**. How does it confirm what you know about William Clowes?

4.4 What was Harvey's contribution to medical progress?

William Harvey (1578–1657) was an English doctor who had studied medicine at Cambridge and Padua. Harvey began work at St Bartholomew's Hospital in London in 1609, and became doctor to King Charles I in 1632. By 1616, he was able to comment in a lecture to medical students: 'The blood must move in a constant circle and is driven by the heart's power.' This was a new theory, different from what doctors had thought for a long time. Yet it was another 12 years before Harvey felt confident enough to publish this theory in his famous book *De Motu Cordis* (On the Motion of the Heart). Why did he take so long to let the world know of his discovery?

Objectives

▶ **Consider** the state of medical knowledge before Harvey's work and the challenge it posed.

▶ **Explain** the methods of and opposition to Harvey.

▶ **Examine** Harvey's achievement and contribution to medical progress in England.

Galen's ideas under attack

According to Galen, new blood was constantly made in the liver, and used as a fuel that was burned up in the body. Galen said that blood passed from one side of the heart to the other through invisible holes. Although this had been challenged by influential doctors such as Ibn al-Nafis (see page 13) and Vesalius (see pages 26–27), they were not believed. In the sixteenth century, other doctors had made important discoveries to do with blood: Realdo Columbo said that blood moved along the veins and arteries, and Fabricius proved there were valves in the veins. William Harvey read what these anatomists at Padua had discovered and built upon their work, but his own theory of the blood directly contradicted the view of the widely respected Galen.

Harvey's theory of the blood

Harvey was a rigorous scientist who had read widely what other doctors before him had written about the heart. From 1616, he set about the exploration of his ideas about blood circulation: he took what he had read as his starting point, then built up his knowledge of the heart through dissection. Harvey studied human hearts, and also observed the slow-beating hearts of cold-blooded animals to understand how the muscles worked. He experimented by trying to pump liquid the wrong way through valves in the veins, proving that blood could only go round one way. He worked out mathematically how much blood would have to be produced if, as Galen said, it was a fuel for the body. Harvey was a careful scientist who drew conclusions from methodical observations and experimentations.

▼ **INTERPRETATION A** *A 1962 painting by Robert Thom, showing Harvey demonstrating how the blood flows one way through the blood vessels of the arm*

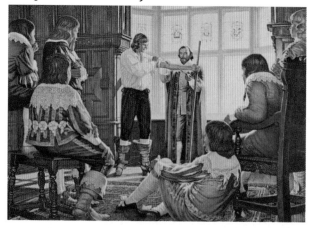

Harvey probably took 12 years from first having the idea of the circulation of the blood to publishing it, because of the revolutionary nature of his theory and also because he did not understand every aspect of how blood works in the body. Even when he published *De Motu Cordis* in 1628, there were still things that he did not know. For example, although he was sure the blood circulated, he did not know why, and he knew that his critics would expect an answer. Neither could Harvey explain why blood in the arteries was a different colour from blood in the veins. He could not tell other doctors how the blood moved from the arteries to the veins, but he suggested that it was absorbed by the veins. Lastly, he knew that if he were right, he would be challenging many of the contemporary medical ideas based upon balancing the four humours, especially the concept of bloodletting.

Fact

In Harvey's lifetime, there was no microscope good enough to see the tiny capillaries that connect the veins to the arteries. In 1661, four years after Harvey died, Professor Marcello Malpighi used one of the first effective microscopes to discover the capillaries. This was proof that what Harvey suggested must be true, and is an example of how technology helped medical progress.

Reactions to Harvey's discovery

When Harvey published his findings in 1628, his critics said he was mad to suggest blood circulated; others ignored his ideas. Some doctors rejected his theory because he was contradicting Galen, who had long been the authoritative voice on how blood worked. They thought that it was impossible that Harvey was correct. Others were very hostile, such as the French anatomist Jean Riolan, at the University of Paris, who called Harvey a 'circulator': this was slang for a travelling **quack** (an unqualified, often useless, doctor). In 1636 in Germany, Professor Caspar Hofmann watched Harvey demonstrate his theory, but then dismissed his calculations about the body's amount of blood as 'the mere trick of an accountant'. Despite all the criticism, Harvey's theory was accepted by many within his lifetime, but it took another 50 years before the University of Paris taught it to medical students.

▼ **SOURCE B** *The title page of Harvey's book, published in 1628*

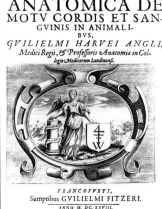

Harvey's discovery was not immediately useful, and further scientific discovery was needed. Doctors would not be able to replace or transfuse blood until 1901, when they knew about blood groups. However, understanding the circulation of the blood was a vital stage in the development of surgery and in the diagnosis of illness. Many modern medical treatments would not work unless blood circulation was understood: for example, blood tests (which help diagnose diabetes or heart, kidney or liver disease), blood transfusions and heart transplants.

Key Word

quack

▼ **INTERPRETATION C** *A nineteenth-century painting showing Harvey explaining to King Charles I the circulation of blood, using the heart of a deer from the royal parks*

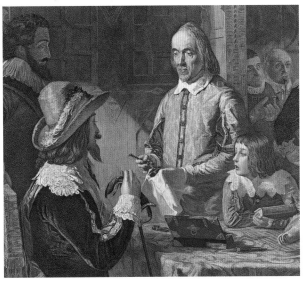

Work

1. What did Galen think blood was for?
2. Describe at least three methods Harvey used in his discovery of how blood works.
3. In pairs or in groups, discuss:
   a. Why did people at the time reject Harvey's theory?
   b. How did Harvey's theories start to be recognised as true?

Practice Question

Explain the significance of the work of William Harvey for the development of surgery.

8 marks

Study Tip

Try to explain whether Harvey's discovery had an impact at the time, and whether it continued to be important later on and to us today.

How scientific was seventeenth- and eighteenth-century medicine?

Although some doctors and surgeons engaged with the Renaissance approach to science and applied lots of rigorous testing in the sixteenth century, many more doctors did not do this. Even in the seventeenth century, ancient unscientific beliefs such as the four humours were still used to treat everyone, from ordinary people to Charles II, the King of England. What kinds of treatments were available at the time? How effective were they?

Objectives

▶ **Describe** traditional and new methods of treating disease in the seventeenth and eighteenth centuries.

▶ **Explain** the ideas behind the traditional or quack treatments.

▶ **Assess** how far the measures were effective.

Treatments fit for a king

At 7:00am on 2 February 1685, King Charles II's excellent health deserted him. One of his doctors, Sir Charles Scarburgh, recorded the detail that the king collapsed with a 'disturbance in his brain'. The royal medical team swung into action. These people were the best that money could buy.

The king received in total some 58 drugs, and he was **purged**, bled, blistered and cauterised. None of these treatments helped the chronic kidney disease that killed him; furthermore, the kidney disease may have been brought about by the poisonous mercury treatments that the king had taken for 'curing' syphilis.

▼ **SOURCE A** *Excerpts from Scarburgh's medical records of King Charles II in February 1685:*

> We opened a vein in his right arm and drew off 16 ounces (425 ml) of blood, then another 8 ounces (212 ml). To free his stomach of all impurities we gave him an **emetic** and then a **purgative** to drain away the humours; to accelerate the purgative we gave him an **enema** and applied blistering agents to his shaved head. (2 February)
>
> We gave him a purgative and drew off 10 ounces (300 ml) of blood from both jugular veins. (3 February)
>
> Alas his Majesty's strength seemed exhausted: he was seized by a mortal distress in breathing, and died. (6 February)

What treatments were available for ordinary people?

Medical treatments available to ordinary people in the seventeenth and eighteenth centuries still depended on what they could afford. They could get medical advice from different people:

- Barber-surgeons: poorly trained people who would give you a haircut and perhaps perform a small operation like bloodletting or tooth pulling.
- Apothecaries: they had little or no medical training, but sold medicines and potions.
- Wise women: their treatments often relied on superstition. However, they often had extensive knowledge of plants and herbs.
- Quacks: showy, travelling salesmen who sold all sorts of medicines and 'cure-alls'.

▼ **SOURCE B** *A seventeenth-century painting of a quack salesman selling medical 'cures' to the sick*

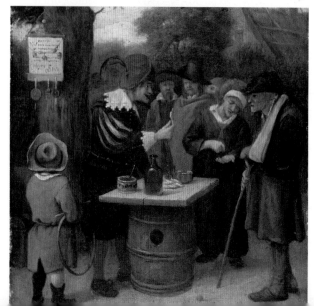

As the treatment of Charles II shows, bloodletting continued to be a common treatment. It was even done regularly to prevent illness. People still had a lot of faith in the royal touch to cure the disease scrofula, or 'king's evil': an average of 3000 people a year arrived in London hoping to be cured by the king's touch. There were many homely herbal remedies that were passed down from generation to generation. Some worked, for example honey can kill bacteria and the willow tree contains aspirin, which dulls pain.

The introduction of the printing press helped ordinary people collect books on herbal remedies, such as the English doctor Nicholas Culpeper's *The complete herbal* (1653). Culpeper used plants and astrology in his treatments. Unusually for the time, Culpeper was highly critical of bloodletting and purging. Along with traditional herbal remedies quack medicine flourished.

▼ **SOURCE C** *In 1659, one of Culpepper's students, William Ryves, published a biography of his master in which he reported Culpeper's view of the Royal College of Physicians:*

> Bloodsuckers, true vampires, who have learned little since Hippocrates, they use bloodletting for illnesses above the waist and purging for those below it. They evacuate and revulse their patients until they faint.

Key Biography

Thomas Sydenham (1624–89)

Sydenham was an English doctor who was famous for recognising the symptoms of epidemic diseases such as scarlet fever, and for classifying illnesses and medicines correctly (such as iron for anaemia). He was critical of quack medicine, and he also stressed the careful observation of symptoms. However, he dismissed the value of dissections and ignored Harvey's discovery because it did not help in treating patients. Sydenham still used all of the usual bleeding methods for treatment, but he often advocated doing nothing and letting nature take its course. His book *Medical Observations* (1676) became a standard textbook.

New lands, new medicines

Explorers on voyages of discovery brought back new natural medicines:

- The bark of the Cinchona tree from South America contained quinine, which helped treat malaria.
- Opium from Turkey was used as an anaesthetic.
- The military surgeon, John Woodall, began using lemons and limes to treat scurvy in 1617.
- Tobacco from North America was wrongly said to cure many conditions, from toothache to plague.

▼ **SOURCE D** *A page from* The complete herbal; *according to Culpeper, the herb lovage (middle left) was 'a herb of the sun, under the sign of Taurus' which strengthened the throat and dried up phlegm*

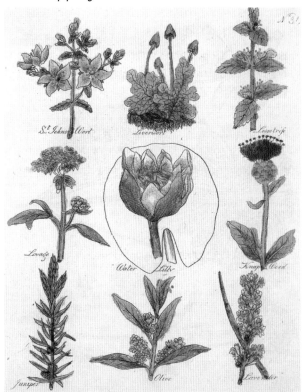

Work

1. What was the theory behind the types of treatment that Charles II received? Explain your answer.
2. Study **Source B**. How did a quack convince people that he or she was to be believed?
3. Make a table of natural and supernatural treatments and remedies used at this time. Highlight the ones that were new.
4. Thomas Sydenham was both innovative and traditional. Do you agree? Why or why not?

How did doctors deal with the Great Plague?

The plague was a devastating disease that hit Britain many times. The best known outbreak was the Black Death in the fourteenth century. There were further, smaller outbreaks of plague over the next few hundred years, and in 1665, it returned once more and killed about 100,000 people in London (around a quarter of the city's population). This time it was known as the Great Plague. It also killed thousands more in the rest of the country. Did people learn anything to help them deal with the latest epidemic of plague?

Objectives

▶ **Explain** how the Great Plague affected people at the time.

▶ **Summarise** the measures taken against the plague.

▶ **Evaluate** how far the measures were scientific.

What did people think caused the Great Plague of 1665?

Many people still believed that the plague was a punishment from God for their sins; other people blamed the movement of planets or 'poisonous' air. The real cause of the plague was again the fleas that lived on rats, which were attracted to the rubbish that was mostly in the poorer parts of the city.

Remedies and treatments at the time had no effect: some patients were bled with leeches. People smoked to keep away the 'poisoned' air, or sniffed a sponge soaked in vinegar. Many strange Medieval remedies that were still used involved using animals such as frogs, snakes and scorpions to 'draw out the poison'. Chickens and pigeons were also used. Treatments that seem odd now were shared as sound medical advice: for example, the apothecary William Boghurst recommended that when close to death from the plague, the remedy to try was: 'You may cut up a puppy dog alive and apply in warm to the sores.'

How did people try to cure the Great Plague?

Doctors still had no cure for the plague. If you were rich enough, one of the simplest remedies was to move to the countryside to avoid catching it. For example, King Charles II and his court left London and moved to Oxford.

There was some evidence that people were beginning to make a strong connection between dirt and the disease. From studying the Bills of Mortality, people realised that most deaths occurred in the poorest, dirtiest parts of the city where people lived in the worst housing.

There was a more organised approach to dealing with the plague this time. Mayors and councillors issued orders to try to halt the spread of the disease. The authorities were concerned with identifying people with the plague, and they paid 'women searchers' who would examine the sick and note those with plague symptoms. Then, the plague victims were quarantined (locked up) in their houses; watchmen stood on guard to make sure that they did not leave and spread the disease. Those houses with plague victims had a red cross painted on the door and the words, 'Lord have mercy on us'.

The bodies of those who had died from the plague were brought out at night when fewer people were about, when the orders to 'bring out your dead' were

▼ **SOURCE A** *A Bill of Mortality showing a list of all the causes of death within London in one week in 1665*

The Diseases and Casualties this Week.			
Abortive	6	Kingfevil	10
Aged	54	Lethargy	1
Apoplexie		Murthered at Stepney	1
Bedridden		Palfie	1
Cancer	2	Plague	3880
Childbed	23	Plurifie	1
Chrifomes	15	Quinfie	5
Collick	1	Rickets	23
Confumption	174	Rifing of the Lights	19
Convulfion	88	Rupture	2
Dropfie	40	Sciatica	1
Drownd two, one at St.Kath. Tower, and one at Lambeth		Scowring	13
		Scurvy	1
Feaver	353	Sore legge	1
Fiftula	1	Spotted Feaver and Purples	190
Flox and Small-pox	10	Starved at Nurfe	1
Flux	2	Stilborn	8
Found dead in the Street at St.Bartholomew the Lefs	1	Stone	2
		Stopping of the ftomach	16
Frighted	1	Strangury	1
Gangrene	1	Suddenly	87
Gowt	1	Surfeit	2
Grief	1	Teeth	
Griping in the Guts	74	Thrush	3
Jaundies	3	Tiffick	2
Impofthume	18	Ulcer	1
Infants	21	Vomiting	1
Killed by a fall down ftairs at St. Thomas Apoftle	1	Winde	8
		Wormes	8

Chriftned {	Males	83	Buried {	Males	2656
	Females	83		Females	2663	Plague 3880
	In all	166		In all	5319

Increafed in the Burials this Week — 1289.
Parifhes clear of the Plague — 34 Parifhes Infected — 96

The Affize of Bread fet forth by Order of the Lord Maior and Court of Aldermen. A penny Wheaten Loaf to contain Nine Ounces and a half, and three half-penny White Loaves the like weight.

Extension

GCSE

Study **Source A** carefully. What are the top three causes of death? What percentage of deaths were due to plague? What do some of the causes of death tell us about medical knowledge at this time?

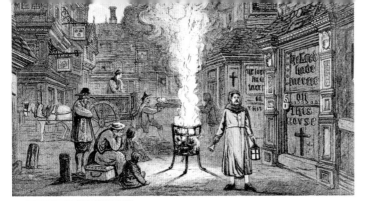

▲ **INTERPRETATION B** *A view of the Great Plague in seventeenth-century London, drawn in 1864*

heard. Bodies were then thrown into carts to be buried in mass plague pits. Fires were lit to try to remove the poisons that were thought to be in the air. Homeowners were ordered to sweep the streets in front of their houses, and pigs, dogs and cats were not allowed in the streets where there was plague. Plays or games that would bring together large crowds were banned. Furthermore, trade between towns with the infection was stopped, and the border with Scotland was closed.

How did the plague end?

It has often been written that the Great Fire of London in 1666 ended the plague because it burned down the poor housing and sterilised the streets by burning the waste. This was not true. The fire destroyed houses within the city walls and by the River Thames. The poorest areas were outside the city walls, where most of the plague deaths happened. The plague actually declined because the rats developed a greater resistance to the disease, and so their fleas did not need to find human hosts. After 1666, quarantine laws prevented epidemic diseases coming into the country on ships.

Work

1 Identify three things in **Interpretation B** that show the impact of the plague.

2 Study **Source C**. Write a description of what you think is happening in each picture.

3 Discuss with a partner: do you agree that the outbreak of the Great Plague was dealt with more effectively than the Black Death? Explain your answer.

Practice Question

Explain two ways in which the Black Death in the fourteenth century and the Great Plague in the seventeenth century were similar. **8 marks**

Study Tip

Identify aspects that are the same, such as knowledge of the cause of the epidemic, measures taken, and the impact at the time.

▼ **SOURCE C** *A broadsheet (news leaflet) from 1665 showing the effects of the Great Plague in a city*

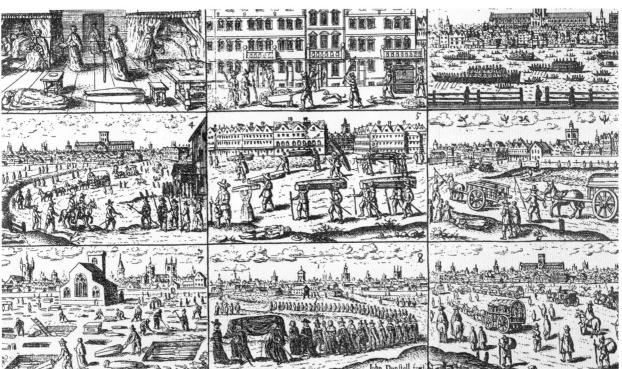

How did hospitals change in the eighteenth century?

5.3

We have seen that Medieval infirmaries or hospitals in England were small and run by the Christian Church: these were places where people came to be cared for rather than to be cured. Many of these early hospitals were funded by rich men donating money to Church causes. However, when King Henry VIII turned England from Catholic to Protestant in the 1530s, his actions affected hospitals. What were hospitals like after the Medieval period? How were they different?

Objectives

▶ **Describe** the changes to the training and status of surgeons and doctors.

▶ **Explain** the growth of new hospitals, and how they were different from Medieval hospitals.

▶ **Assess** the contribution that eighteenth-century hospitals made to medical care.

As part of the religious conflict between Henry VIII and the Catholic Church, the king seized the wealth of rich Catholic monasteries and closed them down (through a process called the dissolution of the monasteries). The king gave money to start hospitals such as St Bartholomew's and St Thomas' in London; it was at St Bartholomew's that William Harvey investigated the circulation of the blood in the seventeenth century.

Who built hospitals in the eighteenth century?

Up to the seventeenth century, hospitals were still places for the sick to rest, to receive simple remedies, and to pray. However, it was in the early eighteenth century that the idea of modern hospitals using modern methods to cure patients began. These hospitals were different because they were founded and supported by the charitable gifts of private people. In London, Westminster Hospital (1719) was founded by a private bank, and Guy's Hospital (1724) was founded by a merchant called Thomas Guy. Guy was a businessman who had initially supported St Thomas' Hospital, but then gave the money to build Guy's. Hospitals were also built by 'private subscription', where local people clubbed together to pay for the construction and running of a hospital.

What happened in an eighteenth-century hospital?

In the new hospitals not only were the sick cared for, but the doctors of the future received training, as medical schools were often attached to hospitals. Individual wards were developed for different types of disease. Although doctors learned mainly through lectures and reading in medical schools, new charity hospitals like the one in Edinburgh gave final-year students the

▼ **SOURCE A** *A drawing of Guy's Hospital from a London guidebook published in 1755*

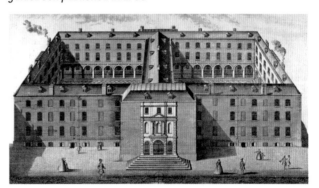

opportunity to gain experience by following the medical professor through the wards.

Doctors also liked to gain an official post at a hospital, because it gave them a better reputation and attracted wealthy private patients. While the doctor attended the ordinary people in the hospital for free, it was the fees paid by private patients which were a doctor's main source of income. The types of treatment given in hospitals were still primarily based on the four humours approach of bleeding and purging. Towards the end of the eighteenth century, as well as treating patients for free, hospitals added dispensaries where the poor would be given medicines without any charge, such as the public dispensary of Edinburgh, which started in 1776.

Types of hospitals

The eighteenth century saw not only general hospitals for the sick, but also specialist types. St Luke's Hospital in London in 1751 became the second large public hospital, after Bethlem, for the mentally ill. London's Lock Hospital for venereal (sexually transmitted) disease opened in 1746.

Hospital	Founded	Paid for by
Royal Infirmary of Edinburgh	1729	Local churches and wealthy citizens
Bristol Royal Infirmary	1735	Wealthy merchant, Paul Fisher
York County Hospital	1740	Gifts from wealthy local people
Middlesex Hospital	1745	Private subscriptions
Manchester Royal Infirmary	1752	Local factory owner, Joseph Bancroft
Addenbrooke's Hospital in Cambridge	1766	Bequest (inheritance) from Dr J. Addenbrooke, and local subscriptions
Leeds General Infirmary	1771	Five local doctors
Birmingham General Hospital	1779	Local businessmen, doctors and landowners

Another new type of hospital was the maternity hospital. For example, wards were set aside in Middlesex Hospital for pregnant women in 1747, and what became known as the British Hospital for Mothers and Babies was set up in 1749.

One particular social problem became more noticeable in the early eighteenth century: high child mortality rates. In the 1720s and 1730s, there were severe epidemics of typhus and influenza, and the death rate among children was alarming. There were poor provisions for babies and children to be given medical treatment. This upset a retired ship's captain, Thomas Coram, who gathered enough public support to build a hospital for sickly or poor children that he 'found' abandoned on the streets. He started the Foundling Hospital in 1741: it cared for orphaned children by giving them a clean environment, clothing and some simple education up to the age of 15. It became one of London's most popular charities.

Hospital boom

Between 1720 and 1750, five new general hospitals were added to London's two ancient hospitals and nine more throughout the country. By 1800, London's hospitals alone were handling over 20,000 patients a year. Compared to 1400, when each of the 470 hospitals in the whole of England had room for only ten patients at most, this was a huge increase. There was a religious motive behind this change in hospital numbers and the focus on patient care and cure. As seventeenth-century conflicts were often based around religion, in the eighteenth century there were some Christians who wanted to include as many different opinions as possible within the Church of England. They downplayed the importance of religious beliefs and styles of church services, and instead stressed that good Christians did more than go to church – they showed their faith by trying to do good deeds in the community.

Attitudes to diseases were changing too. People began to abandon the idea that illness was a punishment for sin; they began thinking that illness could be dealt with from a more evidence-based, scientific point of view. For example, St Luke's Hospital's senior doctor at the time, William Battie, advocated that mental illness was no less curable than any other disease.

▼ **SOURCE C** *A painting of Thomas Coram, by the famous artist William Hogarth, 1740*

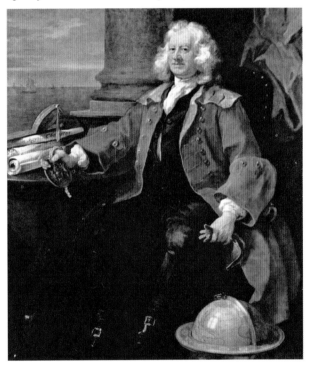

Work

1 What types of people founded hospitals in the eighteenth century?

2 Other than caring for the sick, what else did eighteenth-century hospitals do?

3 What was new about hospitals at this time?

4 Discuss in pairs or in a group: why had attitudes to hospitals changed? In what ways did religion affect hospitals?

Why should we remember John Hunter?

John Hunter was born into a farming family in East Kilbride, near Glasgow, in 1728. At the age of 20, he joined his elder brother William in London, who had started an anatomy school there and was a popular doctor who specialised in childbirth. William's profitable practice meant he had little interest in research but his younger brother John, on the other hand, soon showed a great talent for precise dissection and anatomical research. John's other job was to rob graves at night to supply bodies for his brother's anatomy school! With these diverse talents, how did John Hunter go on to make great changes in the field of anatomy?

Objectives

▶ **Outline** the work of John Hunter.

▶ **Examine** John Hunter's approach to surgery and anatomical knowledge.

▶ **Evaluate** John Hunter's contribution to medical progress.

Look through the following diagram carefully and read about John Hunter in the Key Biography. You can then evaluate his contribution to medical progress.

Key Biography

John Hunter (1728–93)

While working for his brother, John Hunter studied with two of England's most famous surgeons: William Cheselden and Percivall Potts. Hunter became an army surgeon in 1760; after three years he left the army to set up a surgical practice in London. In 1768, he became a surgeon at St George's Hospital. He was appointed Surgeon to King George III in 1776, and Surgeon-General to the army in 1790. Although he earned large amounts of money during his life, he used most of it for research and for his specimen collection. He died in debt and in poverty in 1793.

▼ **INTERPRETATION A** *John Hunter*

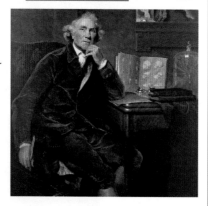

Teaching

Hunter was admitted to the Company of Surgeons in 1768, after which he set up a large practice and trained hundreds of other surgeons in his scientific approach. Many young surgeons that Hunter trained and inspired became great medical teachers and professors, and helped to bring about famous teaching hospitals in nineteenth-century Britain and America. For example, Edward Jenner (see pages 40–41), trained with him and became a firm friend.

Books

Hunter's writings on his scientific research were widely read, and were a major contribution to surgical knowledge. His books helped the surgical profession by showing the theoretical knowledge about anatomy that every surgeon needed. His writings were all based upon his observations, his practical skill as a dissector, and his willingness to experiment. In 1771, he published *The Natural History of the Teeth*, which made use of the dentistry he had learned. His book *On Venereal Disease* (1786) was partly based upon his own self-experimentation; it was translated into several European languages and was widely read. His experience in the army contributed to his book *Blood inflammation and gunshot wounds*: although this was published after his death, it finally put to rest the idea that gunshot wounds were poisoned and therefore that the area around the wound needed to be cut out. Hunter further explained his new idea that the wound should not be made larger, but treated as any other wound. From dissecting many human bodies, Hunter was able to make discoveries about the nature of disease, infections, cancer, and the circulation of the blood.

Scientific method

John Hunter was an early promoter of careful observation and the use of the scientific method in surgeries. He even went so far as to experiment on himself in 1767. There was a debate in his time about whether gonorrhoea and syphilis were the same venereal disease (they are actually different diseases). It was thought that two diseases could not exist together in the same organ of a body. So, Hunter injected himself with pus from the sores of a gonorrhoea patient. Unfortunately, and unknown to Hunter, the gonorrhoea patient also had syphilis. It took him three years to recover using the standard mercury treatment.

Hunter's willingness to try radical approaches was also shown in 1785 when a man was admitted to St George's Hospital with a throbbing lump (aneurysm) on his knee joint. The usual treatment would be to amputate the leg above the throbbing tumour. Hunter's dissections led him to think that if the blood supply were restricted above the aneurysm, then it would encourage new blood vessels to develop and bypass the damaged area. Hunter first tested his theory by experimenting on animals. He then conducted surgery on the patient: he cut into the man's leg and at several points tied off the artery to restrict the blood flow above the aneurysm. Six weeks later the man walked out of hospital: Hunter had saved the man's leg.

What were John Hunter's contributions to medical progress?

Specimens

Hunter collected a huge selection of anatomical specimens. In his collection he preserved 3000 stuffed or dried animals, plants, fossils, diseased organs, embryos, and other body parts. Hunter experimented with inflating narrow blood vessels with wax to study blood flow. A famous item in Hunter's collection was the skeleton of a 2.3-metre-tall (7-feet-7-inches-tall) Irish giant, Charles Byrne, which he acquired in 1783. His collection, including Byrne's skeleton, was later given to the Royal College of Surgeons in England.

Fact

Royal College of Surgeons

Henry VIII allowed the Company of Barber-Surgeons to be formed in 1540, which maintained barber-surgeon standards and controlled qualifications to the trade. By 1745, surgeons were anxious to have their skills recognised as superior to that of barbers, and an Act of Parliament created a separate Company of Surgeons, with a base near to Newgate gaol (to allow the continuous supply of executed prisoners for dissections). The king named the Company of Surgeons as the Royal College of Surgeons in 1800; it still exists to this day to oversee surgeons' training, and to advise the government.

Work

1 Study **Interpretation A**. In what ways did the artist try to show the different achievements of John Hunter's life?
2 a Draw a simple timeline of Hunter's life, and label key events.
   b Using your timeline, explain how each aspect of Hunter's work was linked to the others. For example, how were his books related to his scientific investigations?
3 Do you think we should remember John Hunter? What was the most important aspect of his work?

Practice Question

Explain two ways in which the work of Andreas Vesalius and John Hunter were similar. **8 marks**

Study Tip

Consider whether Vesalius produced work in the same four areas as John Hunter. Who had to overcome the greater opposition to his work?

6.1 How did Edward Jenner help defeat smallpox?

One of the biggest killer diseases in the eighteenth century was smallpox. It was a highly infectious **virus** that passed from one person to another by coughing, sneezing or touching, and it killed 30 per cent of those who caught it. The first symptoms were fever, headache and a rash, followed by pus-filled blisters covering the entire body. Even if you survived, you could be left blind or with deep scars. Doctors at the time tried to prevent smallpox by using **inoculation**, but it was controversial and didn't always work. However, a country doctor named Edward Jenner found a better way to prevent smallpox. How did people react to his discovery?

Objectives

▶ **Describe** smallpox and its treatment using inoculation.

▶ **Explain** how Edward Jenner made his discovery, and the opposition he faced.

▶ **Evaluate** the impact of vaccination.

What was inoculation?

In Medieval China and other parts of Asia, people had been using a basic form of inoculation to prevent smallpox. They scratched pus or scabs from a smallpox victim onto healthy people's skin: they didn't realise it but it gave them a mild dose of the disease, which allowed them to build up resistance against attacks of the full, killer form of the disease. In 1721, smallpox inoculation was in demand in Britain when a fashionable aristocrat named Lady Mary Wortley Montagu had her children inoculated. She had seen it done in Turkey.

Inoculation became very profitable. For example, in the 1760s, a father and son surgeon team, Robert and Daniel Sutton, devised an easier way of inoculation and earned a fortune. Only the rich could afford the treatment though. By the end of the 1770s, more and more doctors used the 'Sutton' method, and it became the normal practice for preventing smallpox. However, there were problems with inoculation:

- There were strong religious objections: some people still argued that God sent illness to test people's faith or to punish them for their sin, so preventing sickness with inoculation was wrong.
- As germs and infection were not understood well at the time, it was hard for people to accept the idea of giving a small amount of disease to prevent a bigger disease. Doctors argued about the risk of dying from smallpox compared with that of dying after inoculation.
- Sometimes inoculation gave people a strong (instead of mild) dose of smallpox, which could kill them.
- Any inoculated person could still pass smallpox to others.
- The poorest people could not afford inoculation, so they were not protected.

However, the practice of inoculation slowly became more common in the 1740s and 1750s.

▼ **SOURCE A** *A painting, from 1823, of a man being shown his face affected by smallpox*

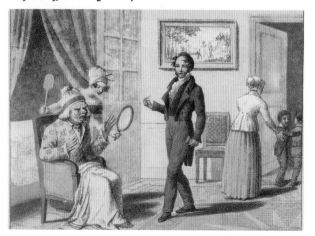

Key Biography

Edward Jenner (1749–1823)

Jenner was an apprentice to a country surgeon from age 13 to 19, then went on to study in London with the renowned John Hunter (see pages 38–39). Hunter encouraged him to conduct experiments and test theories. He returned to Gloucestershire as a country doctor in 1772. In 1798, he published a book on **vaccination**. He was honoured by being appointed physician extraordinary to King George IV in 1821.

Jenner's discovery of vaccination

Smallpox inoculation was a well-known treatment before Edward Jenner became a surgeon. Jenner may have heard stories that milkmaids who caught cowpox (a similar, but milder version of smallpox that commonly affected cows) were protected against smallpox, and he decided to test this theory out.

In Gloucestershire in 1796, Jenner carried out an experiment: he inserted cowpox into a poor eight-year-old boy. If the cowpox worked, then the child would not react to the follow-up smallpox inoculation; if it failed, then he would develop smallpox scabs in the normal way. Six weeks later, he gave the boy smallpox inoculation: no disease followed.

Jenner called his cowpox inoculation technique vaccination, based on the Latin word for cow (*vacca*). To prove that vaccination against smallpox worked without the need for someone to catch cowpox directly from a cow, Jenner gave cowpox to another patient, and then took cowpox pus from that patient to vaccinate a new patient. He tested this 16 times over several weeks. None of the patients reacted to smallpox inoculation, which allowed Jenner to conclude that cowpox protected humans from smallpox.

Opposition to change

Jenner published his vaccination findings in 1798, but he could not explain how vaccination worked, which made it difficult for others to accept it. Many doctors profited from smallpox inoculation, so they disliked his findings. In the London Smallpox Hospital, William Woodville and George Pearson carried out tests using cowpox, but their equipment was contaminated and one of their patients died, so they concluded that Jenner was wrong, and that there was little difference between smallpox inoculation and vaccination. Also, Jenner was not a fashionable city doctor, so there was snobbery

against him. Despite criticisms Jenner had powerful supporters, especially when members of the royal family were vaccinated, and parliament agreed to give Jenner £10,000 for his research in 1802.

Impact of Jenner's discovery

Attitudes changed as people eventually realised that vaccination was more effective and less dangerous than inoculation. Although a few other people had used cowpox to prevent smallpox before Jenner, he had a greater impact because he proved his theories using scientific methods and carefully identified the cowpox disease. Jenner may not have discovered vaccination, but he made others notice it. By the 1800s, doctors were using his technique in America and Europe, and in 1853, the British government made smallpox vaccination compulsory.

> **Work**
>
> 1 In your own words, explain the difference between inoculation and vaccination.
> 2 What were the objections to inoculation and vaccination?
> 3 Prepare an essay plan for the question: 'Explain the significance of vaccination in the development of medicine.'

> **Practice Question**
>
> Has the role of the individual been the main factor in the development of medicine in Britain since Medieval times?   **16 marks**
> **SPaG: 4 marks**

> **Study Tip**
>
> You could refer to Jenner and his vaccination, but there are other people that you could mention. What were these people's special talents? Don't forget you need to consider other factors as well.

How was pain conquered?

By 1800, the status of surgeons had improved, thanks to men like John Hunter (see pages 38–39). However the experience of surgery for the patient was still terrifying. This was because surgeons had no effective way of controlling and stopping pain during an operation. Surgeons managed to solve this problem in the nineteenth century. How did they do it, and did it revolutionise surgery?

Objectives

▶ **Explore** the development of anaesthetics, including the role of James Simpson and chloroform.

▶ **Explain** the opposition to anaesthetics and how it was overcome.

▶ **Assess** the impact of anaesthetics on surgery.

▼ **SOURCE A** *A painting from the seventeenth century showing a foot operation being carried out before anaesthetics were available*

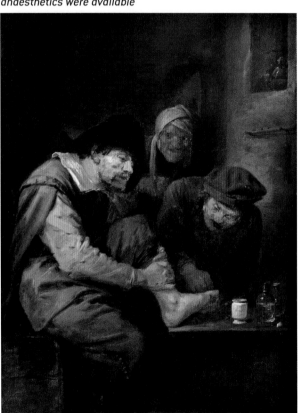

Pain relief was not new: pain-deadening substances were used in the Medieval period. The most important of these were hashish, mandrake, and opium: while these chemicals (made from plant extracts) did dull the pain, it was difficult to judge an effective dose from a lethal one. There was, of course, alcohol, but this made the heart beat faster and the bleeding more difficult for surgeons to control. Some patients had religious objections to alcohol and preferred to sing hymns and suffer the pain. The result was that before surgeons had

an effective and safe anaesthetic, they had to operate quickly to spare the patient pain, and they could not carry out complicated, internal surgery.

Nitrous oxide

As scientific knowledge developed in the eighteenth century, chemists found new anaesthetic substances. The first of these was nitrous oxide. In 1795, the Bristol physician Thomas Beddoes and his young assistant, Humphry Davy, experimented with inhaling nitrous oxide. Davy published an account in 1800: he described how the gas made him laugh, and feel giddy and relaxed, but he did not recognise its medical value. It became a fairground novelty: people paid to inhale it and then fell about, laughing hysterically, much to the amusement of the crowd. It was not until 1844 that an American dentist, Horace Wells, saw fairground laughing gas as an anaesthetic possibility and used it in the removal of one of his own teeth. However, his demonstration failed to convince doctors.

Ether

Around the same time William Clark, another American dentist, experimented with a different chemical: ether. In January 1842, he used it in a tooth extraction. This time doctors took notice. In March, an American country doctor, Crawford Long, used ether to remove a neck growth from a patient. On 16 October 1846, William Morton helped give a public demonstration in a Boston hospital. News of the American anaesthetic experiments quickly spread to Europe. Britain's most acclaimed surgeon, Robert Liston, was keen to be the first to try ether as an anaesthetic. He called it a 'Yankee Dodge' and used it in a leg amputation leg in December. An effective anaesthetic had arrived.

But ether had its drawbacks: it was difficult to inhale, it caused vomiting, and it was highly flammable. For convenience, and to avoid hospital infection, many patients chose to have their operations at home in front of an open fire: using ether in these circumstances could be disastrous.

Chloroform

There was still a need for a safe and effective anaesthetic. The breakthrough came in 1847 when a Scottish doctor, James Simpson, discovered chloroform. The story goes that Simpson and friends had been testing a number of different substances when somebody knocked over a bottle of chloroform. Simpson's wife brought them dinner but found them all sleeping peacefully.

Why was there opposition to anaesthetics?

It seems strange today that doctors should object to using anaesthetics, but some surgeons were used to operating quickly and on a conscious patient. A few army surgeons during the Crimean War (1853–56) thought that soldiers should dutifully put up with the pain. In the early days of

using chloroform, some patients died. This was because men and women of different sizes needed different amounts of chloroform. The most famous case was Hannah Greener, who died in 1848 during an operation to remove her toenail. There were also religious objections to removing the pain of childbirth with anaesthetics, as it was thought to be God's will and a punishment for sin.

However, these objections were quickly overcome by a royal example. By 1850, Queen Victoria had had many difficult labours. Dr John Snow convinced her husband, Prince Albert, that anaesthetics were safe. On 7 April 1853, Snow used chloroform to help Queen Victoria give birth to Prince Leopold. The Queen was in no doubt when she wrote, 'the effect was soothing, quieting and delightful beyond measure'.

For the patient, the conquest of pain was a major step forward, but in itself the introduction of anaesthetics did not revolutionise surgery. This was because there was still a severe death rate from infection (known at the time as 'hospital fever' or 'hospitalism') after the operation. It would take another decade before hospital infections were defeated.

▼ **INTERPRETATION B** *A drawing from the 1860s of Hannah Greener's death from a chloroform overdose during an operation*

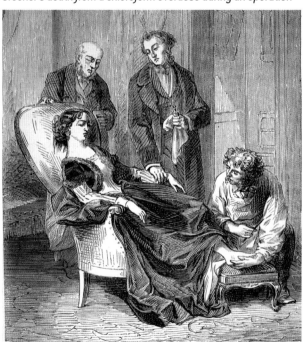

Work

1 a Draw a mind-map to show the different reasons why some people objected to using anaesthetics.
  b Why were the objections overcome?

2 Explain why the development of anaesthetics did not completely revolutionise surgery in the 1840s and 1850s.

3 Write a paragraph of no more than 250 words to explain the contribution of the following individuals to the development of anaesthetics: Humphrey Davy, James Simpson, John Snow, Robert Liston.

Practice Question

How useful is **Source A** to a historian studying the development of surgery? **8 marks**

Fact

Dr John Snow, well known for his work on cholera (see pages 58–59), was one of the first to calculate the correct dosages for ether and chloroform in his book *On Chloroform and other Anaesthetics* (1858).

Study Tip

You could first consider what you can see in the picture. Try to organise your thoughts around the following four headings: pain, infection, bleeding, and operating theatre.

How did doctors in Britain find out that germs caused diseases?

Hospital infections made surgery highly dangerous, but in the 1860s, the new science of bacteriology (study of **microbes**) helped scientists to understand the real causes of infection. How did scientists in Europe and Britain discover that germs caused diseases? Did this discovery help to revolutionise surgery?

Objectives

▶ **Explain** beliefs about causes of infection before the 1860s.

▶ **Describe** the wider public health debate in early nineteenth-century Britain.

▶ **Summarise** Pasteur's experiment and theory.

We now know that an infection is the invasion of the body by microbes (very tiny organisms which include bacteria); different microbes can cause different diseases. But long before scientists made the connection that microbes were actually germs, surgeons believed that when a person was weak, sepsis (or 'poison') began inside the wound and caused it to be infected. They mistook infections for chemical reactions, and didn't realise that they were actually caused by living organisms. They were puzzled about why some deep wounds could heal quickly, while other surface scratches proved to be fatal. Surgeons would initially try to keep the patient healthy and let them heal naturally; then they tried to reduce inflammation with bandages and cleanliness. If the wound became infected, they used cauterising or acids to burn away the affected tissues.

What did people think caused infections?

In 1677, the first basic microscope was invented, which allowed scientists to see the tiny organisms moving about in water droplets, food, and animal and human body parts. Scientists even identified microbes in the blood of sick people, but no link was made between microbes and diseases then. Scientists carried out more experiments, but it did not make things any clearer. For example, in 1699 Francesco Redi boiled up a liquid and sealed it against the air. No microbes appeared, so he concluded that infection came from the outside. However, in 1748 John Needham repeated Redi's experiment and found microbes. People did not realise that the results depended on how clean the equipment was and how careful the scientist was.

In the eighteenth century, scientists had all sorts of ideas about how diseases came about. One theory was **spontaneous generation**: the idea that microbes could appear as if by magic when something rotted. They thought the disease caused the microbes, not the other way round. There was also an assumption that all microbes were much the same.

In the nineteenth century, some people began to question these theories. They believed in **specificity**: that microbes were not all the same, and that certain ones (bacteria or germs) actually caused specific diseases. Scientists found evidence for this. For example, in 1835 Agostino Bassi linked a specific microbe (a fungus) to a silkworm disease called muscarine. In 1840, a Swiss Professor of Anatomy, Friedrich Henle, was the first person to challenge spontaneous generation and suggest microbes were the cause of infection. Henle based his work on Bassi. At the time this new theory was dismissed.

Public health debate about epidemics

In early nineteenth-century Britain, there was increased concern about infection and disease as a result of the surge in epidemic diseases in the fast-growing, dirty, overcrowded industrial towns (see Chapter 9). Public health reformers like William Farr and Florence Nightingale argued that cleaning up the environment would stop epidemics. These people were **anti-contagionists**: they believed that epidemics such as cholera, plague and typhoid were caused when infections interacted with the environment (soil or water) and created the disease that would then attack the weak. Their solution was to clean up an area.

The same ideas were applied by doctors like James Simpson, who wanted hospitals relocated or rebuilt. For example, there were public campaigns to move hospitals such as Manchester Royal infirmary or St Thomas' in London into the countryside. Linked to this debate, many people believed in the popular theory of **miasma**, or 'infectious mist': the idea that there was 'bad air', and that disease was spread by this air.

Set against them were the views of **contagionists**, such as John Simon, who believed that infection was spread by contact with an infected person or bacteria. Contagionists thought that epidemics could be controlled by quarantine or preventing contact. Even though contagionists were correct, the problem for them was that some people who came into contact with a diseased person did not become sick.

The first surgeon in Britain to suggest a non-chemical cause of infection was Thomas Wells in 1864. He referred to the French scientist, Professor Louis Pasteur's recent discoveries, and to the idea of using **antiseptic** substances to destroy microbes.

Who was Louis Pasteur?

The biggest challenge to the theory of spontaneous generation and miasma in Europe came from Pasteur. From 1857 to 1860 he investigated why wine and beer often went sour. He designed a clever series of experiments to show that if air was kept out of the swan neck of a flask, the liquid inside it would not go off. Pasteur identified the specific microbe responsible for souring wine, and showed that heating it to the right temperature

Key Words

microbe   spontaneous generation   specificity
anti-contagionism   miasma   contagionism
antiseptic   Germ Theory

could kill all the microbes. He proved that germs did not come alive on their own, that they could be found in places they could reach easily, and that they infected things and turned them bad. Pasteur concluded that bacteria, or germs, were the real cause and that it was a biological, not a chemical, process. This was Pasteur's **Germ Theory**.

In the late 1860s, largely through the work of the surgeon Joseph Lister, Pasteur's Germ Theory came to the attention of British doctors.

▼ **A** *Pasteur's swan-necked flask experiments*

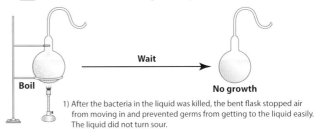

Boil   Wait   No growth

1) After the bacteria in the liquid was killed, the bent flask stopped air from moving in and prevented germs from getting to the liquid easily. The liquid did not turn sour.

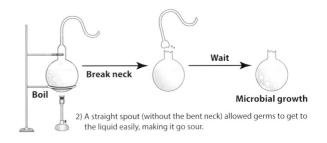

Boil   Break neck   Wait   Microbial growth

2) A straight spout (without the bent neck) allowed germs to get to the liquid easily, making it go sour.

Key Biography

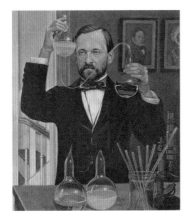

Louis Pasteur (1822–95)

Pasteur was a French chemist and biologist best known for his new discoveries on the causes and preventions of diseases. In 1861, he published his Germ Theory of diseases. He also made important contributions to advances in vaccination, fermentation and pasteurisation (the process of killing bacteria in liquid food such as milk or wine).

Work

1 How did surgeons deal with infection before the 1860s?

2 What were the two main points of view on the public health debate in nineteenth-century Britain?

3 In your own words, describe:
   a Pasteur's swan-necked flask experiment
   b Germ Theory.

How important was Joseph Lister?

Joseph Lister is credited with helping to bring Pasteur's Germ Theory to acceptance in Britain. He also made use of the Germ Theory in his discovery of antiseptic surgery. What was Lister's contribution to medical science?

Objectives

▶ **Describe** Joseph Lister's antiseptic ideas and techniques.

▶ **Assess** why there was opposition to Lister's antiseptic approach in Britain.

Key Biography

Joseph Lister (1827–1912)

Born in Essex, Lister studied surgery and became a fellow of the Royal College of Surgeons in 1852. In 1860, he moved to Glasgow to become a Professor of Surgery. He introduced new principles of cleanliness in surgery.

In Glasgow, 1860, Joseph Lister realised that operations went well as long as the wound was kept free from infection. A Professor of Chemistry, Thomas Anderson, then suggested to Lister that he might be interested in a report by the French scientist Louis Pasteur. Lister thought that Pasteur's Germ Theory might explain the problems of infection he encountered. He asked Anderson if there was a chemical that could kill bacteria; Anderson recommended the use of carbolic acid.

Lister and the antiseptic approach

Lister believed that infections only happened when the skin was broken, and microbes could get in and start an infection. In place of the skin, Lister decided to put a chemical barrier. His first experiment with an antiseptic method was in August 1865. A young boy, Jamie Greenlees, had been run over by cart, which had fractured his leg. The bones were sticking through the skin of Jamie's leg. The traditional surgical procedure would be to amputate above the fracture. Instead, Lister set the bones and used dressings that had been soaked in carbolic acid. The dressings stayed in place for four days, after which time Jamie complained of irritation. Lister feared the worst and expected to find an infection when he took off the dressings. He was impressed to see instead that the fracture and the skin were healing well; the irritation was because of the strength of the carbolic acid. The dressings were replaced and the wound stayed infection-free. After six weeks, Jamie walked out of hospital.

Lister began to test this antiseptic approach out on other surgeries: his method was to spray carbolic acid to coat the surgeon's hands, the wound and the instruments used in an operation. He also soaked the bandages, ligatures and dressings to be applied to the wound in diluted carbolic acid.

▼ SOURCE A *An operation in Edinburgh, 1871, where Lister's methods are being used*

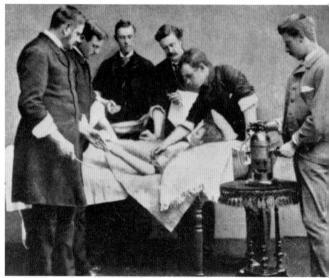

▼ B *The number of patients dying after Lister used his antiseptic method fell dramatically, as his own records show*

Years	Total amputations	Lived	Died	Mortality (%)
1864–66 (without antiseptics)	35	19	16	46
1867–70 (with antiseptics)	40	34	6	15

Reactions to Lister's work in Britain

Lister published his results in March 1867, giving details of 11 patients with compound fractures, none of whom died of infection. He also publicised Pasteur's Germ Theory through his explanation of the antiseptic technique. In August 1867, Lister lectured doctors about his techniques for using carbolic acid dressings in compound fractures. What was controversial was that he said that infection in wounds was caused by microbes in the air. Surgeons had long debated whether to leave wounds open to the air or to cover them with bandages. Lister argued that the oxygen in the air was irrelevant: it was the microbes in the air that were important. He said that the cause of sepsis came from outside the body and not from spontaneous generation, and recommended his form of antiseptic surgery, which people nicknamed 'Listerism'.

But Lister's ideas were criticised. In 1860s Britain, when people were still not very familiar with Germ Theory, Lister's biologically-based theory of infection was not seen to be the correct view. The wider public health debate was still focused on various chemical theories about causes of infection. Many British surgeons were coming up with new theories: for example, in 1868, Professor John Bennett argued that as cells died, they spontaneously generated infection.

The most influential writer on surgical infection was Charlton Bastian, who strongly championed spontaneous generation. He wrote and lectured widely against Listerism in the late 1860s to the early 1870s. And although Lister clearly linked his techniques with Pasteur's proven new ideas, he retreated from these wider discussions about infection theories, and focussed his research on surgery itself.

Reasons for opposition to antiseptic surgery

- Doctors at the time did not accept Pasteur's Germ Theory and there were many opinions in Britain about the role of microbes in surgery and the causes of infected wounds.
- In the late 1860s, antiseptic chemicals had been widely used, and what Lister was proposing was not revolutionary.
- Lister claimed that his methods of dealing with wound infections were superior to others, but some surgeons thought that their existing methods worked perfectly well.
- His methods were often difficult or unpleasant to use. Carbolic acid made people's hands dry up and crack, and breathing it irritated their lungs. It took a long time for the nurses to prepare his carbolic methods. Lister tried to improve his techniques and made changes. Some surgeons pointed to this as a weakness and suggested that Lister did not know what he was doing.

Although Lister gave advice to prevent hospital infections, he still did not fully understand microbes. In the early 1870s, he believed that microbes were very simple things and incorrectly thought that there might be only one type that caused disease. He also did not scrub his hands before surgery, but merely rinsed them in carbolic acid, and he continued to operate in his street clothes.

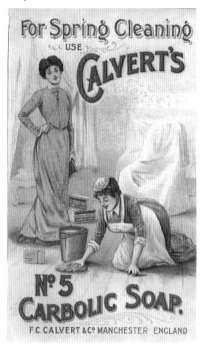

▼ **SOURCE C** *Due to Listerism, carbolic acid became associated with a germ-free environment, as this 1910 soap advertisement shows*

Work

1 Describe Lister's antiseptic techniques in surgery.

2 Explain how Lister applied Pasteur's Germ Theory to his own discoveries.

3 Why was there opposition to Lister's antiseptic ideas?

Practice Question

Explain the significance of Lister's work for the development of medicine. **8 marks**

Study Tip

Consider the impact of Lister's work at the time in saving lives and changing the way surgeons and doctors thought about their work. Mention the use of antiseptics in medicine today.

The debate continues in Britain: accepting Pasteur's Germ Theory

By the 1890s, surgeons in Britain had moved away from antiseptic methods of surgery to **aseptic** ones. So, surgical practices became safer, but doctors were still unsure how people got infections. Various infection theories were still hotly debated, despite Lister's attempts to share Pasteur's Germ Theory with the British audience. Why did it take so long for Pasteur's work to be accepted in Britain? What were the steps towards the acceptance of Germ Theory in Britain?

Aseptic surgery

By the 1890s, surgeons in Europe and North America went beyond Lister's antiseptic methods and developed aseptic surgery. Operating theatres were no longer to be soaked in carbolic acid in order to kill microbes; rather, microbes were to be excluded from the start. Surgeons had to be well-scrubbed, wearing gowns and new, thin flexible gloves, and using well-sterilised instruments. The first British surgeon to use rubber gloves was Berkeley Moynihan in the 1890s. Facemasks, rubber gloves, surgical gowns, and replacing huge public operating theatres with smaller rooms dramatically reduced infections. Aseptic surgery depended on accepting Pasteur's theory. When did this begin to happen in Britain?

The evidence for Germ Theory

Louis Pasteur understood from his experiments that specific germs might turn liquid foods – such as milk – sour, or give diseases to animals. However, his ideas were not immediately accepted in Britain. Also, most doctors at the time still did not believe that microscopic germs could harm something as large and advanced as a human. Instead, the idea that specific germs might cause diseases was first noted in Britain not by doctors, but by vets.

The cattle plague of 1866

During the cattle plague of 1866, it was assumed that the disease had started spontaneously. Farmers were reluctant to kill cattle, so the disease quickly spread nationwide. It was soon realised that the outbreak could only be controlled by the quarantining and slaughtering of cattle. As a result of this, there were food shortages and prices rose.

The government appointed the leading scientific user of the microscope, Professor Lionel Beale, to investigate the crisis. In June 1866, Beale's findings not only recognised the specific microbe responsible, 'a living particle of extremely minute size', but also demonstrated how the microscope could help with complex medical research. The cattle plague was clearly identified as an example of a contagious disease.

▼ **SOURCE A** *A public notice in 1867 in Eccles, Berwickshire showing the use of quarantine to control the cattle plague*

CATTLE PLAGUE.
NOTICE.

NOTICE IS HEREBY GIVEN, That persons who are not employed on the Farm of LANGRIG, in the Parish of Eccles and County of Berwick, are prohibited from entering any Building or Enclosed Place on said Farm, without my permission in writing.

JOHN DOVE.

LANGRIG,
19th November, 1867.

NOTICE IS FURTHER GIVEN, That any person contravening this Order is liable, under the Act of Parliament 29 Vic. cap. 15, to a Penalty of £5, or imprisonment for each offence, and the Police are authorised to apprehend offenders, or report them for prosecution.

GEORGE H. LIST,
Chief Constable.

COUNTY POLICE OFFICE,
Dunse, 19th November, 1867.

J. M. WILKIE, PRINTER DUNSE.

Bastian versus Tyndall

Despite Beale's findings, the dominant view in Britain about infection was still that it occurred spontaneously, and that it was a chemical action that produced poisons. The views of Charlton Bastian, Professor of Anatomy at University College London, dominated debate and he had written many articles in the late 1860s that supported spontaneous generation.

However, in January 1870, Bastian came up against the arguments of the physicist John Tyndall. Tyndall very publicly defended Pasteur's Germ Theory, and argued against Bastian. Tyndall lectured on both dust and disease, bringing together Pasteur and Lister's work with experiments on light that showed the tiny microbes in ordinary air.

Typhoid fever

Many British doctors' views about Germ Theory finally changed due to public health debates about the disease typhoid fever. Typhoid fever was an infectious bacterial fever, and symptoms included red spots and severe

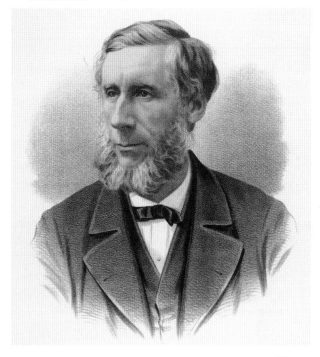

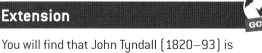

intestinal irritation. It was common throughout Britain, but public awareness was raised in 1861 when it was said to be the cause of Prince Albert's death. Anti-contagionists had always said that typhoid fever was the disease that clearly proved they were right about cleaning up urban areas. Therefore it was important news when, in 1874, the scientist Emanuel Klein announced that he had identified the typhoid microbe. Immediately, Tyndall criticised spontaneous generation and said that Germ Theory explained typhoid fever. Unfortunately, Klein was mistaken: he had not found the typhoid microbe.

However, within two years, the work of Robert Koch and others after him proved to doctors that Germ Theory could explain human diseases such as typhoid fever.

Fact

Natural remedies

While debates raged about whether illnesses were caused by biological or chemical processes, many doctors continued to use natural drugs, such as herbs, to heal people and prevent sickness. For example, it had been known since the seventeenth century that Peruvian bark could prevent malaria.

Work

1   How does aseptic surgery differ from antiseptic surgery?

2   a   How did the 1866 cattle plague contribute to people's acceptance of Pasteur's Germ Theory in Britain?

    b   What about typhoid fever? How did that contribute to the acceptance of the theory?

3   It took a long time for Germ Theory to be accepted in Britain. Create a timeline or a chart to explain the contribution of all the individuals who helped in its acceptance, and the opposition they faced at the time. Make sure you include: Lionel Beale, John Tyndall, Joseph Lister.

Extension

You will find that John Tyndall (1820–93) is an important figure in public health debates in Britain in the nineteenth century. Research his contributions to nineteenth-century science.

How did scientists discover that germs caused human diseases?

Louis Pasteur made a momentous breakthrough in 1861 with the publication of his Germ Theory. He had proven that germs were all around, and some of them could cause disease – but he was a chemist, not a doctor. He wasn't able to link his Germ Theory to humans. Many doctors did not realise that germs could harm humans too. It took a German doctor, Robert Koch, to apply Pasteur's theories to human diseases. How did Koch's work impact on medical progress in Britain?

Objectives

▶ **Describe** Robert Koch's methods and discoveries on microbes.

▶ **Evaluate** the contribution of Koch to medical progress.

▶ **Explain** Koch's impact in Britain.

Key Biography

Robert Koch (1843–1910)

Dr Robert Koch was born in Germany. He studied to be a doctor, and was a brilliant student under Professor Frederick Henle (the first person to challenge spontaneous generation and suggest that microbes caused infection). Koch worked as a surgeon in the Franco-Prussian War; from 1872 to 1880 he was German Medical Officer. He was a pioneering microbiologist, and he was appointed to the Imperial German Health Bureau in Berlin. Koch is known as the founder of modern bacteriology (study of bacteria), and made key discoveries in public health, including identifying the specific bacteria that caused anthrax, cholera, and tuberculosis. He was awarded the Nobel Prize in 1905.

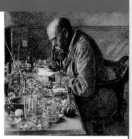

Koch and Pasteur's Germ Theory

Koch first became famous in 1876 for his work on anthrax microbes. Anthrax is a disease that causes sores on the lungs, and can kill both humans and animals. Koch found a way of staining and growing the particular germ he thought was responsible for anthrax. He then proved that it was this bacterium that caused the disease by injecting mice and making them ill. For the first time, he was able to apply Pasteur's theory to prove that germs caused diseases in humans.

Later on, using similar methods, Koch was able to identify the germs that caused the deadly diseases of cholera and tuberculosis. Although Koch was very much inspired by Pasteur, they saw each other as rivals: through their new scientific discoveries, they competed in honour of their respective countries.

Robert Koch's methods

Koch not only made improvements, but also changed the study of bacteria. Previously it was believed that most germs were the same. His methods and findings allowed other scientists to locate specific germs that might cause specific human diseases. Some of his main principles of studying bacteriology follow.

- To prove a specific bacterium was responsible for a specific disease, Koch said the bacterium had to be present in successive experimental animals that were infected with it. The bacterium could be retrieved from each dead animal and cultured (grown) again.

- Koch developed the technique of growing microbes on a plate made of solidified agar (a seaweed extract), which encourages microbes to grow.

- He found ways of using dyes to stain specific microbes under the microscope so that they would stand out among all the other germs.

- He also developed ways of photographing microbes so that other scientists could study them in detail, and find them in samples.

Koch turned bacteriology into a science. He perfected the methods that allowed scientists to hunt specific disease-causing microbes.

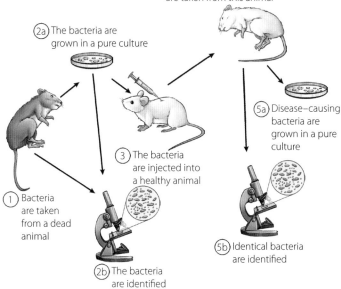

▼ **A** *Robert Koch's laboratory method of identifying specific disease-causing microbes*

④ The disease affects the second animal; bacteria are taken from this animal

②a The bacteria are grown in a pure culture

⑤a Disease–causing bacteria are grown in a pure culture

③ The bacteria are injected into a healthy animal

① Bacteria are taken from a dead animal

⑤b Identical bacteria are identified

②b The bacteria are identified

Koch didn't work alone – he had a team working with him, and also trained many young scientists to use his methods. Scientists produced a string of discoveries in the decades to follow, identifying the specific germs responsible for typhoid, pneumonia, meningitis, plague and tetanus.

Reactions to Koch's and Pasteur's work in Britain

Role of Tyndall

As the debate about typhoid rumbled on in mid-1870s Britain (remember that Emanuel Klein thought he had identified the typhoid bacterium in 1874, but was mistaken), Germ Theory was finally starting to win acceptance. Firstly, a number of British germ studies were published between 1873 and 1875: these used microscope evidence and answered many questions about germs. For example, in 1874, William Dallinger and John Drysdale published a paper describing the life cycle of microbes. Secondly, John Tyndall continued to promote Pasteur's Germ Theory widely, and in 1876, he lectured to British doctors on Koch's discoveries about anthrax.

Roberts and Cheyne

In the end, it was the crucial contributions of two British doctors that won over opinion about Germ Theory in Britain. A Manchester doctor, William Roberts, who had supported Tyndall's criticisms of spontaneous generation, developed a doctor's version of the Germ Theory of disease: he linked all the laboratory research work with the practical evidence of surgeons and public health doctors. In particular, he used the work of Koch to draw attention to germs and their role in human infections.

Then, in 1879, Joseph Lister's deputy surgeon, William Cheyne translated Koch's work into English. He also wrote a paper based on Koch's findings. Cheyne explained that some microbes present in healthy tissue and wounds were harmless and did not always produce disease.

By the 1880s, British doctors accepted Germ Theory and its role in explaining infection. Surgery and public health benefited from Germ Theory, but doctors dealing with disease deep inside the body could not use intense heat or powerful antiseptics. Nobody had yet come up with a way to kill or alter microbes in the body without damaging healthy tissue. Despite this, there was great optimism that, as more specific microbes were isolated and identified, appropriate **vaccines** would follow.

Practice Question

Explain two ways in which the work of Pasteur and Koch were different.

8 marks

Study Tip

Consider how much change each scientist brought about in medical thinking. You could refer to how many lives were affected by their work.

Work

1 Explain some of Koch's principles in your own words.

2 Discuss in groups or in pairs: in your opinion, which was the more important achievement of Robert Koch – his discoveries, or his methods? Why?

3 Add the contributions of William Roberts, William Cheyne and Robert Koch to your timeline from Work question 3, page 49.

4 Who was most responsible for the acceptance of the Germ Theory in Britain? Explain your answer.

The search for vaccines and cures in Europe and Britain

As more specific disease-causing germs were identified, many doctors and scientists were eager to produce vaccines for the diseases. The two great giants of bacteriology – Louis Pasteur and Robert Koch – fought to make the next breakthrough.

Objectives

▶ **Summarise** Pasteur's and Koch's work in the 1880s.

▶ **Explain** the factors involved in the search for vaccines between 1800 and 1900.

Pasteur and Koch were not the only ones making scientific discoveries in the second half of the nineteenth century, but they were the most famous. There were several main factors that contributed to scientific breakthroughs in the 1880s and 1890s, as seen through the rivalry of Pasteur and Koch.

1 War

1871: The rivalry between Pasteur (a Frenchman) and Koch (a German) increased after France had lost a war against Germany. At this time, nations were interested in medical research because armies could lose more men to illness than to bullets. Defeating diseases could have a big impact on the battlefield.

2 Government and finance

Both Pasteur and Koch were equipped with a laboratory and a team of scientists, paid for by their governments. They both were recognised internationally with many honorary awards and prizes, including the Nobel Prize in 1905 for Koch, and the Copley Medal in 1874 for Pasteur.

3 Individual character

Pasteur: 1860s: He was a determined and hardworking scientist, despite suffering a stroke and losing his daughter to typhoid.

1871–75: He returned to work and continued to investigate agricultural problems, studied the fermentation of beer, and defended his ideas about Germ Theory.

1876–81: Koch's success in identifying the anthrax germ in 1876 spurred Pasteur and his team on to quickly develop vaccines for two animal diseases: cholera and anthrax.

Koch: 1882: Koch was also a strong-minded and rigorous scientist and doctor. After his first discovery, he went on to study tuberculosis (TB). The rivalry was further inflamed when Koch made a great breakthrough in 1882 by identifying the TB germ.

1883: Koch's team of scientists also beat a French team to identify the cholera germ.

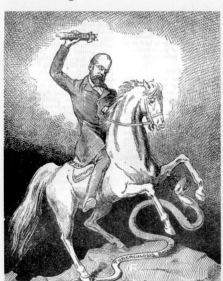

KOCH AS THE NEW ST. GEORGE.

Fact

TB was the largest cause of adult deaths in Western Europe. Throughout the 1870s, it killed over 50,000 people a year in Britain.

◀ **SOURCE A** *A cartoon from the 1880s; it shows Koch conquering the bacteria responsible for tuberculosis*

4 Luck

1879: Pasteur was investigating chicken cholera, a disease that was crippling the French poultry industry. By accident, Charles Chamberland, one of Pasteur's assistants, used an old and weakened sample of the disease microbes. When the chickens were injected, they survived. More importantly, these chickens also survived when they were then injected with fresh strong germs. Pasteur showed that the weakened microbes built up the chicken's own defences against the stronger ones. This was how vaccines, or the prevention of diseases, worked!

5 Communication

Pasteur developed a vaccine against the deadly animal disease anthrax. He demonstrated his vaccine in front of an audience of politicians, farmers and journalists in France in May 1881. News of this success was quickly sent around Europe by electric telegraph. News of Koch's discoveries was spread by scientific articles and at conferences.

6 Teamwork

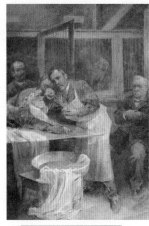

1880–84: Working with Charles Chamberland and Pierre Roux, Pasteur developed a vaccine for rabies, based on the dried spinal cords of infected rabbits. But he was reluctant to test it on a person.

1885: Pasteur proved that vaccines worked on human, as well as animal, diseases when he gave a boy who had been bitten by a rabid dog the rabies vaccine.

▲ **INTERPRETATION B**

Pasteur and his team collecting the saliva from a rabid dog

1888–90: The rivalry continued over research on diphtheria, a highly contagious disease that affects the nose and throat. In France, Pierre Roux, one of Pasteur's scientists, showed that the diphtheria germ produced a poison or toxin. In 1890 in Germany, Emil Behring, one of Koch's students, showed that weakened diphtheria germs could be used to produce an antitoxin.

Impact of Pasteur's and Koch's work in Britain

Between them, Pasteur and Koch encouraged a whole new generation of scientists to study deadly diseases and to find ways of preventing them.

Many of these discoveries soon spread to Britain. For example, Joseph Lister introduced the French serum for diphtheria to Britain, and it was widely used after 1895. Within 10 years, the mortality rate in England dropped to less than half.

Fact

As well as the search for biologically-based vaccines to prevent illnesses, scientists also tried to find chemicals that would attack the specific germs that caused illnesses, and cure them. In 1909, Paul Ehrlich (a German doctor who had been part of Koch's team), developed the first chemical cure for a disease: he found that the chemical Salvarsan 606 cured syphilis. He described it as a 'magic bullet', because it targeted the harmful germ specifically, and destroyed it without harming the rest of the body.

Work

1. Why did governments pay for scientific research?
2. **Source A** shows admiration for Koch's achievement. How do you know?
3. Explain the contributions of the following people to the development of effective treatment for diseases: Pierre Roux, Emil Behring, Paul Ehrlich.
4. How did Pasteur's discoveries help people understand how vaccinations worked?

Practice Question

Was luck the main factor in the development of vaccines between 1880 and 1900? **16 marks**

SPaG: 4 marks

Study Tip

Write about luck and choose two other factors you think were important.

How dirty were Britain's towns in the early 1800s?

Public health – the health and well being of ordinary men, women and children – was in a poor state in 1800s Britain. The average age of death for a working man was about 30 years of age. In some places, such as Liverpool, it was 15! In Manchester, one in every five children died before their first birthday and one in three died before they reached the age of five. In fact, despite improved medical knowledge and understanding, people's health in general may even have been worse in the early 1800s than in earlier centuries. What happened to public health at that time? Why was it in crisis?

The growth of towns and cities

Britain's towns and cities grew very quickly in the first 50 years of the 1800s, and the health of the people living in them grew steadily worse. For example, Sheffield had a population of just 12,000 people in 1750, but by 1850, the number had risen to over 150,000. People had flocked to Sheffield for one simple reason: to get a job in one of the new factories, and the promise of the new life that went with it. Many new factories were built in the north and midlands of England in the early 1800s, and needed thousands of workers to operate the machinery that made cloth, pottery, iron or steel. And as a single factory alone might employ hundreds of people, rows of houses were built quickly, 'back-to-back'.

▼ **B** *A plan of back-to-back housing in Nottingham, 1845*

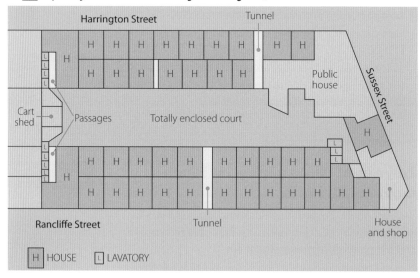

▼ **A** *The population of British towns and cities, 1801–51*

Town	1801	1851
Bradford	13,000	104,000
Glasgow	77,000	329,000
Liverpool	82,000	376,000
Birmingham	71,000	233,000
Manchester	70,000	303,000
Leeds	53,000	172,000
London	957,000	2,362,000
Bath	33,000	54,000
Norwich	36,000	68,000
York	17,000	34,000

▼ **SOURCE C** *Late nineteenth-century back-to-back housing in Staithes, Yorkshire*

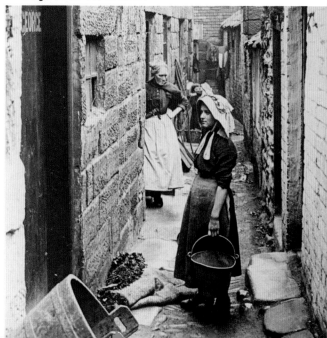

These squeezed as many workers as possible into each street. Almost all the houses were crowded, often with five or more people living in one small room. In 1847, 40 people were found sharing one room in Liverpool.

Disease in the slums

Few of the houses had toilets. The best some families could manage was a bucket in the corner of the room that would be emptied now and again, into the street, or stored outside the door until there was enough to sell to a farmer as manure. Occasionally, there was a street toilet (a deep hole with a wooden shed over it) but this would be shared by lots of families. Sometimes a water pump provided water, but often the water only came from the local river or pond, and this would be as filthy as the water in the streets.

There were no rubbish collections, no street cleaners or sewers, and no fresh running water. Sewage trickled down the streets and into nearby rivers, yet most families washed their clothes, bathed in and drank from the same river. It was little wonder that terrible diseases like typhoid, tuberculosis and cholera were common. No one really knew how people caught diseases, or how to avoid catching them.

A government response?

Governments in all major European nations were concerned about the outbreaks of serious disease in their towns and cities, but were unclear as to how to deal with them. A link had been made between the poor conditions in Britain's towns and cities and the rising death rate, but in the early 1800s people still did not know what really caused disease, so there were no clear strategies to deal with it.

▼ **SOURCE D** *From a report on the 'Prevalence of Certain Physical Causes of Fever' (1838) by the doctors Neil Arnott and James Kay:*

> In Glasgow, which I first visited, it was found that the great mass of the fever cases occurred in the dirty narrow streets and courts, in which, because lodging there was cheapest, the poorest naturally had their homes. Seven hundred and fifty four of about 5000 cases of fever which occurred in the previous year were from one such locality, between Argyle Street and the river.
>
> We entered a dirty low passage like a house door, which led from the street through the first house to a square court immediately behind, which court, with the exception of a narrow path around it leading to another long passage through a second house, was occupied entirely as a place to keep dung.

▼ **E** *Some of the most common diseases of the 1800s*

Disease	Cause	Description
Typhoid	Contaminated water or food	Spread by poor sanitation or unhygienic conditions; sewage would get into the water supply that people drank
Tuberculosis (TB)	Germs passed in the air through sneezing or coughing	Spread rapidly in crowded conditions; another type of TB was caused by infected cows' milk
Cholera	Contaminated water or food	Several cholera epidemics swept the country in the early 1800s

Work

1 Define 'public health'.

2 Give as many reasons as you can why it was so easy for disease to spread in cities in the early 1800s.

3 Look at plan **B**.
   a Copy the plan of back-to-back houses in your notebook.
   b What is missing from these houses that we take for granted today?
   c On your plan, mark which house (or houses) you would least like to live in. Give reasons for your choice.

Extension

Back-to-back housing was built in many towns and cities all over Britain. By the mid-twentieth century, most of it had been knocked down. Identify a town or city near you and try to find out about its back-to-back housing. Where was it? When was it built? Who lived there? When was it knocked down? What is built there now? Note: some back-to-back housing still exists. In Birmingham, for example, it is preserved as a 'living museum' (see www.nationaltrust.org.uk/birmingham-back-to-backs).

Fighting one of Britain's deadliest diseases: cholera

In the early nineteenth century, disease spread quickly in filthy, overcrowded cities such as Leeds, Liverpool, Bradford and Manchester. But people at this time didn't understand that germs caused their illnesses. Far away in laboratories, scientists like Louis Pasteur had started to make the connection, but down in the streets and slums of Britain, people continued to live their lives and get their filthy water in the same ways as they had always done. And then, in 1831, a new and frightening disease arrived in Britain: cholera. What was the impact of this deadly disease, and how did the government react?

Objectives

▶ **Examine** the main cholera epidemics of the nineteenth century.

▶ **Explore** the role of public health reformers.

▶ **Assess** the impact of local and national government initiatives to improve public health, including the 1848 Public Health Act.

Cholera: the first outbreak

In 1831 alone, cholera killed around 50,000 people. Victims were violently sick and suffered from painful diarrhoea; the skin and nails turned black just before the victim fell into a coma and died. So many people were dying that cemeteries had to be closed because they were too full: bodies had started to poke through the ground's surface, letting off a disgusting stench. One vicar in Bilston, West Midlands, even wrote that 'the coffins could not be made fast enough for the dead'.

What frustrated many was the complete lack of understanding of this new killer disease – there was no cure. People knew of diseases that killed more people than cholera, but this was something they hadn't experienced before, and it struck with such devastating speed, killing thousands in a few days.

▼ **SOURCE A** *A Dudley Board of Health poster, from the 1840s, announcing the burial procedure for people who had died of cholera*

CHOLERA.

THE

DUDLEY BOARD OF HEALTH,

HEREBY GIVE NOTICE, THAT IN CONSEQUENCE OF THE

Church-yards at Dudley

Being so full, no one who has died of the
CHOLERA will be permitted to be buried
after *SUNDAY* next, (To-morrow) in either
of the Burial Grounds of *St. Thomas's*, or
St. Edmund's, in this Town.

All Persons who die from CHOLERA, must for the future
be buried in the Church-yard at Nethertor.

BOARD of HEALTH, DUDLEY.

What did people think caused cholera?

Many people at this time commonly believed disease was spread by miasma: an 'infectious mist' given off by rotting animals, rubbish and human waste. This led some towns to clean up their streets. But the importance of clean water still wasn't understood. The cholera epidemic passed after a few months and life was getting back to normal. Some thought that cholera would never return.

Action at last

After more outbreaks of cholera in 1837 and 1838, the national government decided to act. In 1839, they set up an inquiry to find out what the living conditions and health of the poor were like all over Britain. The man in charge was a government official named Edwin Chadwick.

Chadwick's report shocked Britain. Over 10,000 free copies were handed out to politicians, journalists, writers and anyone who could change public opinion. Twenty thousand more were sold to the public.

It didn't really matter that Chadwick mistakenly believed in the miasma theory: what was important was that the report highlighted the need for cleaner streets and a clean water supply. And it showed that most people were wrong in thinking that the poor were to blame for bad housing and living conditions. In fact, there was little they could do about it; it was parliament who would have to do something to improve public health.

▼ SOURCE B *A drawing from the 1830s showing barrels of tar being burned on the streets of Exeter; the smell from the tar was thought to stop the miasma spreading cholera along the street*

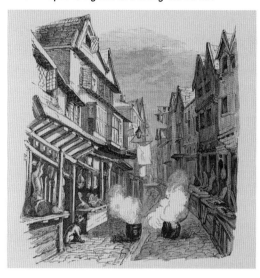

Key Biography

Edwin Chadwick (1800–90)

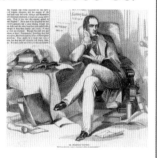

Chadwick was a lawyer who devoted his efforts towards health and social reforms. Over a two-year period, he worked on his famous public health inquiry by sending out doctors to most major towns and cities; they set questionnaires and interviewed hundreds of people. The results of the report were published in 1842.

▼ SOURCE C *Excerpts of conclusions of Chadwick's 1842 report on the 'Sanitary Conditions of the Labouring Population of Great Britain':*

Disease is caused by bad air and these diseases are common all over the country.

The bad air is caused by rotting animals and vegetables, by damp and filth, and by overcrowded houses. When these things are improved, the death rate goes down.

A medical officer should be appointed to take charge in each district.

More people are killed by filth and bad ventilation each year than are killed by wars.

People cannot develop clean habits until they have clean water.

The poor cost us too much; the rich pay to feed and clothe orphans. Money would be saved if fewer parents died of disease. A healthier workforce would work harder too.

The poor conditions produce a population that doesn't live long, is always short of money, and is brutal and rough.

Work

1 Why do you think cholera was one of the most feared diseases of the 1800s?

2 Look at **Source B**. Why are these people burning tar in the streets?

3 Read **Source C**.
   a Make a list of changes Chadwick wanted to make.
   b What evidence is there that Chadwick believed in the miasma theory?
   c Do you think Chadwick felt sorry for the poor? Explain your answer carefully.

Practice Question

How useful is **Source C** to a historian studying public health problems in industrial Britain?   **8 marks**

Study Tip

Write about what the report says and the person writing it. Say why he was well placed to comment on conditions.

Extension

Chadwick's report showed that the length of people's lives was greatly affected by where they lived. The table below shows the average age of death for different classes of people in two different places. Give reasons for the differences between and within classes in different areas.

	Leeds (town)	Rutland (country)
Upper class	44	52
Middle class	27	41
Working class	19	38

Fighting one of Britain's deadliest diseases: cholera

Cholera returns

A lot of people paid attention to Chadwick's pleas for improvements, but the government didn't do anything. In the 1800s, many people thought politicians had no right to meddle in the private lives of citizens. This attitude was known as **laissez-faire**, French words meaning 'leave alone': the government should not interfere in the lives of ordinary people and force them to change. These people said it was the government's job to keep law and order, not to keep people clean. And some Members of Parliament were making vast fortunes from rents in the slums; tearing the slums down and rebuilding them would cost them money!

But cholera changed their minds. As news reached Britain of another cholera epidemic sweeping across Europe, the government decided to act at last, and passed a Public Health Act in 1848.

▼ **D** *The main points of the 1848 Public Health Act:*

> A 'Central Board of Health' is to be created in London. This is a group that will work to make any improvements that might improve public health.
>
> They can force some areas to set up their own 'Local Board of Health' where there is a high death rate, or where more than ten per cent of ratepayers ask for one. These boards will have the power to appoint a specialist Medical Officer, provide sewers, inspect lodging houses and check food quality which is offered for sale.

The act gave local town councils the power to spend money on cleaning up their towns, but this was not compulsory. Some towns, such as Liverpool, Sunderland and Birmingham, made huge improvements. However, many others didn't bother to do anything. By 1853, only 103 towns had set up their own Boards of Health, and in 1854 the Central Board of Health was closed down because of strong resentment of government interference.

▼ **SOURCE E** *Adapted from the Liverpool Health Committee, 1849, listing what needed to be done in the city; 'water closets' were simple holes in the ground, covered by a small shed, which collected human waste; 'privies' were much healthier because they contained a seat, with a bucket underneath, which was removed and emptied by the local council on a regular basis:*

> The substitution of water closets for privies, the abolition of cesspools, the banishment of all toxic factories from inhabited areas, the removal of slaughterhouses, an abundant supply of water, and widening of streets.

Dr John Snow's discovery

Meanwhile, the plague of cholera continued. In 1848, 60,000 people died of cholera; 20,000 died of it in 1854. During the 1854 epidemic, a doctor named John Snow made a major breakthrough in proving there was a link between cholera and water supply.

The discovery that cholera was a water-borne disease (a disease carried in water) was a remarkable achievement. The government now had a growing batch of evidence about

Key Biography

John Snow (1813–58)

Snow was a famous surgeon who worked in Broad Street, Soho, London. In 1854, over 700 people living in this street, or in nearby streets, died of cholera within ten days, so Snow began to investigate. Through meticulous research, he found that all the victims in this small area got their water from the Broad Street water pump. Those who didn't die seemed to be getting their water from other places. Snow asked permission to remove the handle of the water pump so people were forced to use another. There were no more deaths in the street! Snow investigated further and found that a street toilet, only one metre from the pump, had a cracked lining that allowed polluted water to trickle into the drinking water. Snow had proved that cholera was not carried through the air like a poisonous gas or miasma. Instead it was caught through contagion: by coming into direct contact with a cholera sufferer; or in this case, drinking some water contaminated by a victim's diarrhoea.

the state of the nation's health within the dirty, overcrowded towns. They even had medical evidence that made a link between cholera and water supply. But the government did not do much about it, until a 'Great Stink' would finally force them into action.

▼ **SOURCE F** *John Snow's map showing cholera deaths (shown as black blocks) between 19 August and 30 September 1854*

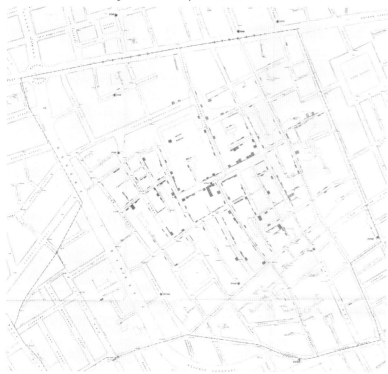

▶ **SOURCE G**

An English engraving from 1866 called 'The Death Dispensary'; it appeared in Fun *magazine, commenting on London's polluted water supply. This magazine was published weekly and contained amusing poems and parodies, as well as sports and travel information and topical cartoons (often of a political nature).*

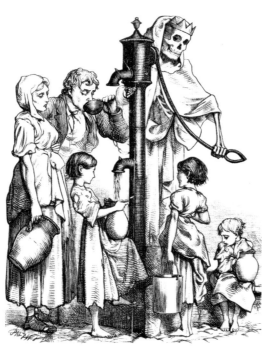

DEATH'S DISPENSARY.

Key Word

laissez-faire

Fact

John Snow used scientific observation to show how cholera spread, but he didn't know why it spread. Louis Pasteur didn't publish his Germ Theory until 1861 (see pages 44–45), which would have helped to explain the results Snow had recorded.

Work

1 a What is meant by the term laissez-faire?
  b Why do you think so many politicians believed in laissez-faire?
2 a List some of the things that Local Boards of Health could do.
  b Why do you think public toilets were far more important in the nineteenth century than they are today?
  c What were the limitations of the 1848 Public Health Act?
3 Imagine you are Dr John Snow. Write a letter to the National Board of Health explaining:
  a how you think cholera is spread (you will need to summarise your evidence)
  b what you think should be done about it.
4 Look at **Source E**.
  a In your own words, explain how Liverpool tried to improve public health in the city.
  b How close were their ideas to those suggested by Chadwick?
5 Look at **Source G**. What point is the person who drew this cartoon trying to make?

9.3 The Great Stink

London in 1858 was a dirty, overcrowded, unsanitary city. Its main river, the Thames, was a dumping ground for human sewage, household rubbish, horse dung, slaughterhouse waste and chemicals from factories. The river water was also used for washing clothes and cooking! Raw sewage could sometimes be seen trickling out of the pumps that pulled water out of underground streams. Despite the fact that Dr Snow had worked out the link between the deadly disease cholera and dirty water supplies, the city streets remained as filthy as ever and were a breeding ground for disease.

Objectives

▶ **Describe** the 'Great Stink' of 1858.

▶ **Examine** the reasons for and the consequences of Bazalgette's sewer system.

▶ **Assess** the impact of public health reform (including the 1875 Public Health Act).

The Great Stink

▼ **SOURCE A** *A Punch cartoon commenting on the state of the River Thames in 1858; 'Father Thames' introduces his children, Diptheria, Scrofula and Cholera, to London*

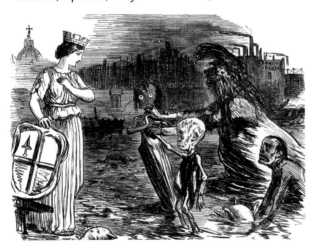

In the summer of 1858, a heat wave caused the filthy River Thames to smell worse than ever. The smell was so bad that the politicians in the Houses of Parliament (right next to the river) demanded to meet somewhere else. Some called it the summer of the 'Great Stink'. The stench from the Thames, combined with Dr Snow's new evidence about cholera, caused such alarm that MPs turned to a man they hoped could save their city. His name was Joseph Bazalgette.

A new sewer system for London

Three years earlier, Bazalgette had been asked to draw up plans for a network of underground tunnels – or sewers – to intercept all the waste from nearly one million London houses before it had a chance to flow into the Thames. The beauty of Bazalgette's design was that it used gravity and the slope of the London river basin to get the sewers to flow downstream towards the sea. At Crossness he built a pumping station where pumps, the largest ever made at the time, pumped the sewage up to the level of the Thames; at high tide, it was released into the river and the river did the rest, taking it out to sea. MPs wanted London's streets free of sewage quickly. Bazalgette was given £3 million (about £1 billion today) in 1858 and told to start immediately. Using 318 million bricks, he built 83 miles of sewers, removing 420 million gallons of sewage a day.

Timeline: Public health reforms

1842	1848	1853	1858	1866	1875
Chadwick Report	First Public Health Act	Compulsory vaccination	Work on London sewer system begins	Sanitary Act: this makes local councils responsible for sewers, water and street cleaning; each town has to have a health inspector	Artisans Dwelling Act (also known as the Housing Act): this makes house owners responsible for keeping their properties in good order; it also gives local councils the power to buy and demolish slum housing if it is not improved

▼ **SOURCE B** *Bazalgette standing, on the right, above a London sewer during construction; many of Bazalgette's sewers are still in use today*

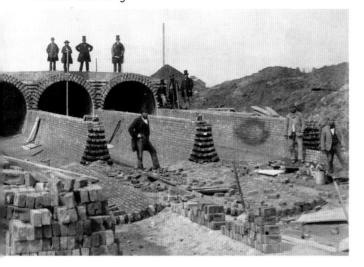

The sewers were finished in 1866, and when fully operational, cholera never returned to London. Soon, parliament went into a flurry of action to improve public health.

Of course, other measures improved life expectancy too, including better nursing and surgery techniques, but the nineteenth century saw government take much more responsibility for the state of public health.

The death of laissez-faire?

In 1867, working-class men living in towns were given the vote. It was these same people who had been suffering most from poor living conditions. Soon, political parties realised that if they promised to improve conditions in the towns, the working-class people living there would vote for them. When the Conservative Party won the general election in 1874, it was largely due to working-class votes. Soon after, they introduced many new public health reforms. Many historians today think that working-class people getting the vote is one of the most important reasons why politicians began to improve the nation's health.

1875	1875
Second Public Health Act: local councils forced to appoint Medical Officers to be responsible for public health; councils are also ordered to cover up sewers and keep them in good condition, supply fresh water, collect rubbish and provide street lighting	Sale of Food and Drugs Act: this introduces guidelines for the quality and sale of food and medicines

Fact

The death rate (the number of people dying per 1000 of the population) fell from about 39 in 1800 to 18 in 1900. The average age of death rose from 30 to 50, and the total population of the country rose from about 10 million in 1801 to 38 million in 1901. So the population increased nearly four times – mainly because people were living longer.

Extension

Study **Source A**. How useful is it to a historian studying the development of public health in Britain?

Work

1. Cholera never returned to London after Bazalgette's sewers were fully operational. Should Bazalgette receive all the credit for this? Explain your answer.

2. Look at **Source B**. What does this photograph tell you about:
   a. the scale of the work involved in building the sewers
   b. the building methods of the time?

3. Design a diagram that explains the improvements made in public health in the nineteenth century. Include information on: diseases, death rates, influential people like Chadwick, Snow and Bazalgette, and government action.

Practice Question

Explain two ways in which a Medieval town and early nineteenth century London were similar.
8 marks

Study Tip

Write about the ways in which clean water and sewage were treated as well as the town authorities' attitudes to public health.

What can a study of penicillin tell us about the development of modern medicine?

A recent exhibition at the British Museum in London estimated that the average number of pills that a person takes in his or her lifetime in the UK is around 14,000! Indeed, the chances are that in recent weeks or months you might have taken a variety of pills for aches and pains. And if you have had an infection, many of you will have been given a drug called penicillin, which was the world's first **antibiotic**. The industry that develops and produces all these drugs for use in medicine and health care is known as the **pharmaceutical industry**. So how did this industry develop? And what can a study of the world's first antibiotic tell us about the development of modern medicine?

Objectives

▶ **Explore** the development of the pharmaceutical industry.

▶ **Outline** the factors in Fleming's discovery and the development of penicillin.

▶ **Assess** the impact of this discovery and development.

Prevention and cure

During the late nineteenth century, knowledge about disease increased greatly. Soon after doctors and scientists started to identify which bacteria caused which diseases, a search began to find ways of preventing people from getting the diseases, and also curing people who already had them. These two lines of research – prevention and cure – led to some dramatic advances in the understanding of health and medicine.

Prevention

When Louis Pasteur published his Germ Theory in 1861, the world began to realise that bacteria were the cause of many diseases; not miasma, or God's punishment, or any of the other causes that people had believed for centuries. And after Pasteur and Robert Koch identified different types of bacteria that caused specific diseases, doctors began to use weakened forms of the bacteria to allow the body to build up immunity to the disease if it struck again. This was something that had been successfully tried – but not understood – by Edward Jenner with smallpox in 1796. Soon vaccines, as they became known, were created to prevent diseases such as diphtheria, TB, rabies and anthrax.

Cure

Koch found that certain chemicals sought out and found specific bacteria in the body. His assistant, Paul Ehrlich, worked at finding a chemical that would not only stain a specific type of bacteria – but kill it too! After Ehrlich's discovery of a chemical cure for syphilis in 1909, other 'magic bullets' were found by scientists over the next 20 years. Most notable was prontosil, a red chemical that worked against the germs that caused blood poisoning. Prontosil's active ingredient was sulphonamide (a chemical from coal tar). More magic bullets or 'sulpha drugs' were soon developed to cure or control meningitis, pneumonia and scarlet fever.

Staphylococcus

By the 1920s, one nasty germ in particular, named staphylococcus, remained undefeated by any magic bullet. It was a highly resistant form of bacteria that had over 30 different strains, and it caused a wide range of illnesses and diseases, especially different types of food and blood poisoning.

However, a way to kill staphylococcus was close at hand. Scientists had known since the 1870s that some **moulds** (yes, the stuff that grows in an unwashed coffee cup or on your wet football boots after a week out in the rain!) could kill germs. One type of mould – penicillin – proved particularly good at killing staphylococcus. Its discovery, and the eventual development of penicillin as the world's first and most famous antibiotic, is a fascinating story. It's a tale of luck, individual brilliance, war, and huge breakthroughs in scientific and technological understanding. As you work through this case study, try to look out for each of the complex factors that contributed to the penicillin story.

Key Biography

Alexander Fleming (1881–1955)

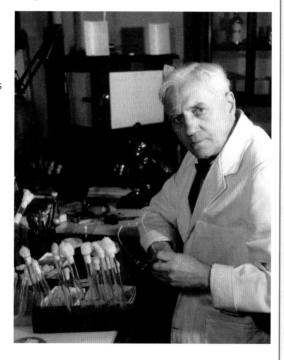

During the First World War, the **bacteriologist** Alexander Fleming was sent by St Mary's Hospital in London to study the treatment of wounded soldiers. Many were suffering from the ill effects of the staphylococcus germ. Ordinary chemical antiseptics, which were not used as much by this time, were not working on some of the deeper wounds and Fleming saw at first hand the agony suffered by the soldiers. In 1928, he published findings on the effects of the penicillin mould. He won a Nobel Prize in 1945 (along with Howard Florey and Ernst Chain) for the 'discovery of penicillin and its curative effect'.

Fleming realised the germ-killing capabilities of penicillin and published his findings that year. Even though we know today that penicillin is an antibiotic, Fleming did not realise this and concluded that it was a natural antiseptic. But the one test that was missing from his work was the test of injecting penicillin into an infected animal. This would have shown that penicillin could be used as a medicine, and could kill infections in the body without harming living cells. The results of such a test would likely have sparked great interest in penicillin and could have advanced its development. As a result, few people regarded Fleming's work as a major breakthrough and gradually even Fleming himself lost interest in it. However, the story didn't end there: soon, other key factors played a role in the success of penicillin.

Fleming's discovery

After the First World War, Fleming became determined to find a better way to treat infected wounds and conducted detailed experiments. By 1928, he was still working on the hard-to-kill staphylococcus germs. When he went on holiday, he left several plates of the germs on a bench. When he came home, he noticed a large blob of mould in one of the dishes. Upon investigation, he noticed that the staphylococcus germs next to the mould had been killed. An excited Fleming took a sample of the mould, and found it to be the penicillin mould. It appeared that a **spore** from a penicillin mould grown in a room below Fleming's had floated up the stairs and into his laboratory.

Fact

An antiseptic is a chemical that is mostly used outside the body, on the skin and on objects, to kill germs. An antibiotic is a medicine that can be digested or injected into the body, and kills certain germs as it travels around the body. Penicillin is an antibiotic.

Work

1   Explain what is meant by the term 'magic bullet'.

2   How was Ehrlich's work different from Pasteur's?

3   Discuss in groups or in pairs: why do you think Fleming is usually thought of as the discoverer of penicillin?

What can a study of penicillin tell us about the development of modern medicine?

The development of penicillin

In the 1930s, a research team from Oxford University began compiling a list of all the natural substances that could kill germs. They got hold of Fleming's article on penicillin and began to get very excited. Two of the scientists, Howard Florey and Ernst Chain, applied to the British government for some money to begin further research into the germ-killing powers of penicillin. They received only £25; not nearly enough to even start their research properly. In fact, they were probably lucky to get £25: the British government, by 1939, was far more interested in the Second World War that had just started. However, Florey and Chain pressed on and, despite the fact that penicillin is extremely difficult to grow and extract (from the mould), they managed to produce enough to successfully test it on eight mice.

Their next move was to test it on humans, but they needed 3000 times the amount they had used on the mice. So, over a couple of months, the two scientists turned their university department into a penicillin-producing factory. Using old milk bottles, hospital bedpans and a bath in which to grow the bacteria, they slowly collected enough penicillin to use on one human.

A 43-year-old policeman, Albert Alexander, was selected because he had been scratched by a rose bush and a nasty infection had spread all over him. All other drugs had failed on him. When he was injected with penicillin, the infection began to clear up. Tragically though, after five days, the penicillin ran out and the patient died; but the success of penicillin had been noted by all involved. The next step was to try to work out how to produce masses of it.

How was penicillin mass-produced?

▼ **SOURCE A** *Penicillin being mass-produced in the 1940s; a worker at Pfizer is shown carefully preparing vials of penicillin solution*

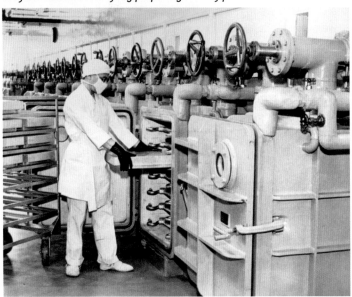

The Second World War was a vital factor in transforming the supply of penicillin. The growing number of soldiers with infected wounds meant that more penicillin was needed – and quickly. In June 1941, Florey went to America to meet with the US government. Realising the lifesaving properties of this new wonder treatment, they agreed to pay several huge chemical companies to make millions of gallons of it. By the start of 1943, enough had been made to treat just 100 patients, but by 1944 there was enough to treat 40,000. By the end of the war in 1945, Britain and the USA were working closely together and enough penicillin was being produced to treat 250,000 people a month. Drug companies began using their production methods to make penicillin for public use as soon as the war ended.

The need to produce huge quantities of penicillin was a key factor in the growth of the pharmaceutical industry. In the early 1800s, drugs and medicines were generally produced by small-scale businesses. However, towards the end of the nineteenth century, some of the larger companies we know today, such as GlaxoSmithKline, Hoffmann-La Roche and Pfizer had begun: they started out as chemists and pill-makers, or producers of chemicals used by scientists. The discovery of penicillin as a 'wonder drug' in the early twentieth century led to huge government-sponsored programmes to develop and produce it.

This meant that the pharmaceutical industry had both the finance and the technology to research and develop medicines for all sorts of diseases. Today, the pharmaceutical industry is one of the biggest in the world, worth an estimated £200 billion to £300 billion and employing nearly 80,000 people in the UK alone.

> **Fact**
>
> Pharmaceutical drug production became industrialised in the late nineteenth century with the growth of pharmaceutical companies and also with new technological advances: for example, the invention of the gelatine pill capsule (1875), and the first tablet-making machine (1843, in England).

The impact of penicillin

▼ **SOURCE B** *A British soldier being treated with penicillin in June 1944*

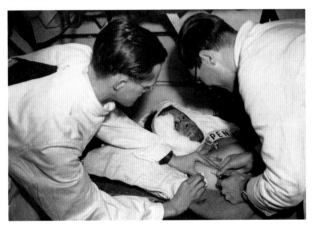

It has been estimated that, during the Second World War, 12 to 15 per cent of wounded British and American soldiers would have died without being given penicillin to fight their infections. Also, thousands of injured soldiers returned to service much quicker than they would have done without penicillin treatment. After the war, penicillin became available for doctors to use as a means of prevention and cure for their patients. It was classified as an antibiotic, and has gone on to save the lives of millions of people. Indeed, unless you have an allergy to penicillin (around ten per cent of people do), almost all of you will probably have been prescribed penicillin by a doctor at some time.

Other antibiotics followed: streptomycin (1944), for example, proved an excellent treatment for tuberculosis, while tetracycline (1953) was great for clearing up skin infections. Mitomycin (1956) has been used as a chemotherapy drug for treating several different types of cancer.

Who gets the credit?

If you were asked on a television game show, 'Who discovered penicillin?' then the answer would almost definitely be 'Alexander Fleming'! This is due to the very well known story of the mould floating into his laboratory and attacking the bacteria on his germ dish. But Fleming certainly didn't develop penicillin, nor was he the first to use it to treat an infection.

So perhaps Florey and Chain should be included in any answer to the question, 'Who developed penicillin?' They were the first to test it directly on a human body, and were the first to develop a way to produce large quantities of the drug. So who does deserve the credit for giving the world penicillin?

> **Work**
>
> 1 Explain the part played in the penicillin story by: Joseph Lister; Alexander Fleming; Florey and Chain; Albert Alexander; the US government.
>
> 2 How was the discovery of penicillin quickened by luck, and by war?
>
> 3 a Explain what is meant by the term 'antibiotic'.
>   b List some of the antibiotics mentioned on these pages. State the approximate dates they were introduced and give an example of the types of disease they fought.

> **Practice Question**
>
> Has science been the main factor in the development of penicillin?
>
> **16 marks**
>
> **SPaG: 4 marks**

> **Study Tip**
>
> Refer to two other factors such as government and the role of the individual.

> **Extension**
>
>
>
> Challenge yourself to do further research on penicillin. Find out about the role of: Norman Heatley; Andrew Moyer; Alfred Richards.

How have drugs and treatments developed since 1945?

Great changes in understanding disease had taken place in the years up to 1945. The government had started to take more responsibility for public health too, including clearing the worst of the overcrowded slum areas of the dirtiest towns and building proper sewer systems. The widespread use of anaesthetics and antiseptics, and now the discovery of the first antibiotics, meant that life expectancy had increased from the age of 46 (men) and 50 (women) in 1900 to just over 60 (men) and 65 (women) in 1945. What were the medical discoveries and developments that happened in the latter half of the twentieth century?

Objectives

▶ **Examine** the key developments in new knowledge about the body and disease, surgery and treatments since 1945.

▶ **Assess** how these developments have been affected by a variety of factors.

The second half of the twentieth century saw an explosion in scientific and medical discoveries and developments that proved significant in achieving a fuller understanding of health and medicine. This resulted in life expectancy levels increasing to around 79 (men) and 83 (women). Indeed, a recent UK government article claimed that one in two babies born today is expected to live until its 100th birthday.

The timeline below charts some of the most significant changes in the fields of knowledge about the body and disease, surgery and treatment.

1950

1960

1950
Canadian surgeon William Bigelow performs the first open-heart surgery to repair a 'hole' in a baby's heart

1952
First miniature hearing aid is produced

First kidney transplant is carried out (the first in the UK is in 1960)

1954
Free vaccine for diptheria, whooping cough and tetanus (the 'triple vaccine') in the UK

1958
First pacemaker is fitted (in Sweden); this is a mechanical device that maintains a regular heartbeat (the first in the UK is in 1960)

1962
Surgeons at a hospital in America re-attach the arm of a 12-year-old boy

1957
The drug thalidomide is developed in Germany; it is used to treat morning sickness during pregnancy but it causes terrible deformities in babies; today it is used in the treatment of AIDS and some cancers

1955
Free vaccine for polio in the UK

1951
Mexican company Syntex develops norethisterone: a human-made hormone that prevents women ovulating; this leads to the production of the first contraceptive pill

1953
American Leroy Stevens discovers stem cells; these are cells in multi-cellular organisms that are able to renew themselves and differentiate into specific cell types

Francis Crick and James Watson map out the **DNA** structure, building on the 1951 work of Rosalind Franklin; this leads to such developments as gene therapy, genetic **screening** and genetic engineering

1964
Free vaccine for measles in the UK

1948
Free vaccine for TB in the UK

1973

British scientist Geoff Hounsfield invents the CAT scanner, which uses x-ray images from many angles to build up a 3D image of the inside of the body

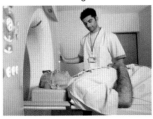

1978

Doctors use IVF fertility treatment to help childless women become pregnant throughout the 1970s, and in 1978, Louise Brown from the UK becomes the first 'test tube baby'

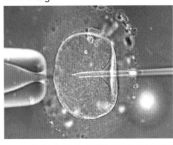

Work

1   Write a sentence or two about the following:
    a   IVF treatment
    b   DNA.

1984

At Harvard University in the USA, two burn victims are given skin grafts; the skin had been grown in a laboratory 'skin farm' from tiny pieces – one square centimetre grew to half a square metre

1969

Free vaccine for rubella (German measles) in the UK

1975

Endoscopes are developed; these are fibre-optic cables with a light source that allow doctors to go into small cuts in the skin to 'see' inside the body

1970

British scientist Roy Calne develops the drug cyclosporine, which prevents the body rejecting transplanted organs

1986

British woman Davina Thompson becomes the first heart, lung and liver transplant patient

1972

British surgeon Sir John Charnley develops hip replacements

1970

1980

1987

MRI scanning is widely used to monitor brain activity, which is especially useful for finding brain tumours or stroke damage

1968

First British heart transplant at Papworth Hospital

1980

After a global vaccination campaign, smallpox is officially declared eradicated; so far, the only human disease where this has been possible

1967

Christian Barnard, a South African heart surgeon, performs the first heart transplant; the patient lives for 18 days (the first in the UK is in 1968)

Fact

DNA (*deoxyribo nucleic acid*) is the material that makes up genes. It is like a long list of instructions, or a code, that operates all the cells in your body. The instructions are grouped together in genes, and each gene has a different function – for example, it might determine your eye or hair colour, or whether you will develop a disease. All genes can be passed from parent to child. A British scientist called Rosalind Franklin, an expert in X-rays, photographed DNA in 1951, capturing the pattern of DNA. This enabled fellow British scientists Francis Crick and James Watson to suggest DNA's double-helix structure. Crick and Watson went on to publicise the mapping of the DNA structure and the fact that genes could pass information from one generation to the next.

How have drugs and treatments developed since 1945?

1996
Researchers in Scotland breed the first cloned animal: a sheep called Dolly, cloned from a cell taken from a six-year-old ewe. Cloning is the process of creating an identical copy of an original organism. Dolly died in February 2003 from a lung disease. The idea of using cloning technology on humans is one of the medical world's most controversial issues

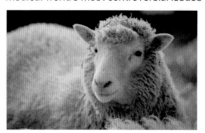

2002
American surgeons implant electrodes connected to a miniature computer into the visual cortex of a blind man; using a video camera mounted onto his glasses, the man is able to 'see' well enough to drive a car

2008
First full face transplant

2020
In the UK, the first COVID-19 vaccine was administered in December 2020 as part of a mass vaccination programme.

2006
First HPV (anti-cancer) vaccine approved

2013
First human liver is grown from stem cells

1990

2000

2010

2020

1990
The **Human Genome Project** formally launches: it is the world's largest collaborative biological research project that aims to decode all the genes in the human body and identify their roles; the money for this international scientific project comes from the governments of the USA, Britain, Japan, China, France and Canada, as well as drug companies that hope to profit from developing drugs based on understanding DNA

2003
The Human Genome Project is declared complete with the final sequencing of the entire human genome, which is a huge breakthrough in understanding how genes help determine who a person is; ongoing research into links between genetics and treating diseases come from the information produced by this project

2006
First partial face transplant is carried out

2007
Huge breakthrough in visual prosthetics (bionic eyes) with the release of the Argus II prosthetic eye

2020
French scientist Emmanuelle Charpentier and American scientist Jennifer Doudna are awarded the 2020 Nobel Prize in Chemistry for their discovery of 'genetic scissors' – a new genome editing technology

Technology

New technologies such as **keyhole surgery** and MRI scanning have helped doctors and surgeons to develop new techniques for identifying illnesses and operating on them. Discoveries, such as understanding more about DNA, have helped gene researchers work out family relationships, trace ancestry, use DNA analysis to solve crimes, and find specific genes involved in diseases. With the ongoing research on the human genetic code (made possible by the Human Genome Project), scientists are optimistic that soon doctors can better understand cancer and lots of other illnesses.

War

Two world wars meant that the government spent a fortune on research and testing so that the latest drugs and surgical techniques were available for wounded soldiers. Doctors had to find better ways to treat casualties too, thus advancing medical knowledge. Sadly, wars and conflict continue to take place and the research, testing and development continue.

Government and finance

Governments spend far more money on research and care than ever before. For example, the British government has a huge breast and cervical cancer screening programme which aims to identify illness before it develops. Drug companies too, spend huge amounts on research and development, hoping to make money from cures.

Communication

New ideas spread rapidly due to the increased use of television, news media and the Internet. Television and radio advertisements have made more people than ever before aware of health risks associated with smoking and alcohol, for example.

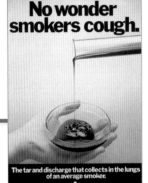

No wonder smokers cough.

The tar and discharge that collects in the lungs of an average smoker.

Change in attitudes

Modern politicians have realised that one of their main priorities is to help and protect the people they serve. In recent years the British government has introduced 'Healthy Eating Standards'. This means that food served in schools must include high-quality meat and fresh fruit and vegetables. Schools cannot serve drinks with added sugar, crisps, chocolate or sweets in school meals and vending machines.

Reasons why drugs and treatments have developed greatly in the late twentieth century

Individual character

As across all periods of history, the late twentieth century saw some geniuses in action: Crick and Watson, and Geoff Hounsfield in Britain, for example.

Extension

Which do you think is the main factor affecting medical progress? Write a paragraph (no more than 250 words) explaining your reasons why. Make sure you mention at least two other factors and why you think they are not the main factors.

Practice Question

Explain the significance of the individual sciences – physics, chemistry and biology – for medical progress in the twentieth century.   **8 marks**

Study Tip

Show how each branch of science has contributed to progress in medical treatments.

Work

1   What is the Human Genome Project?

2   Imagine you have to choose three medical developments from the twentieth century to include on a web page entitled 'The greatest advances in medical history'. Which three developments would you choose? Give reasons for your choices.

3   a   In your own words, explain how medical progress has been affected by:
    • government and finance
    • technology
    • war
    • individual character
    • communication.

    b   Can you find examples on the timeline on pages 66–68 that match these factors?

Beyond mainstream medicine

Researchers predicted in 2002 that by 2070, people would live to the average age of 100 (it stood at 80 for women and 75 for men at the time the prediction was made). They put this down to the advances made in medicine in the twentieth century. So what happens if people develop immunity to prescribed drugs? How do things like '**positive health**' and '**alternative medicines**' fit into all this?

Objectives

▶ **Define** antibiotic resistance.

▶ **Describe** alternative treatments.

▶ **Explore** advances in healthcare in the latter half of the twentieth century.

Antibiotic resistance

The battle against disease, and other causes of death, continues in the same way as it always has. The range of new drugs being produced every year is huge. Drug companies spend billions of pounds on research, knowing that enormous profits can be made. Since the development of penicillin, there have been many more discoveries of different types of antibiotics that kill all sorts of bacteria, including tuberculosis; and lots of different vaccines that prevent and control diseases such as polio, measles, mumps and whooping cough.

However, despite the development of new drugs, not all drugs work: even proven antibiotics can fail. In fact, the effectiveness of antibiotics can lead to their overuse, prompting bacteria to evolve and become increasingly resistant to common antibiotics. An example of an antibiotics-resistant bacteria is called MRSA (methicillin-resistant Staphylococcus aureus), first reported in a British study in 1961.

▼ **A** *Causes of death in the UK, 1919 and 2000*

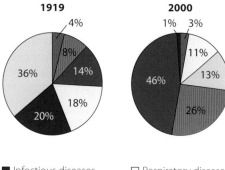

1919
4%
8%
14%
36%
18%
20%

2000
1% 3%
11%
46%
13%
26%

■ Infectious diseases (whooping cough,TB)
■ Heart/circulatory diseases
▨ Cancer
□ Respiratory diseases (pneumonia/bronchitis)
▨ Nervous system
■ Injuries/poisoning

Alternative treatments

Doctors are still not able to cure some diseases, such as viruses like AIDS and the common cold. Cancer –

although treatable depending on the type – is still a major killer disease. As a result some people turn to alternative therapies to find ways of improving their health and treating their illnesses.

Alternative medicine is the term used to describe any other way of treating an illness or health condition that doesn't rely on mainstream, doctor-dispensed scientific medicine, or on proven evidence gathered using the scientific method. It includes a wide range of practices and therapies.

▼ **B** *An extract from a survey on the popularity of alternative therapies, in which 2000 British people took part*

Alternative therapy	Tried by (%)	Satisfied (%)	Not satisfied (%)
Herbal medicine	12	73	18
Homeopathy	4	66	16
Acupuncture	3	50	47
Chiropractic	2	68	19
Hypnotherapy	2	43	50

Those in favour of alternative medicine argue that these treatments consider the patient as a whole, instead of beating a disease down by finding the cause and then hitting it with drugs. However, some have put the increase in popularity of alternative healthcare down to a lack of confidence in conventional doctors and hospital care. In Britain in the 2000s, a number of scandals (such as that concerning Dr Harold Shipman, who murdered his patients and stole their money) reduced public confidence. However, generally speaking, satisfaction levels with the treatment people get from their hospitals and GPs remains high. A 2014 survey of nearly 2000 people found that 71 per cent were satisfied with the service they received from their doctor.

Since the 1980s, alternative medicine has become more and more popular in Britain, and some of it (such as acupuncture) is now available on the NHS. In fact, a

Aromatherapy

What is it? Aromatherapy is the use of essential oils from flowers, fruits, roots and leaves. The oils are inhaled or massaged into the skin.

Effect? The inhaled scents are said to stimulate particular parts of the brain, which promote healing, while massaged oils pass into the bloodstream and can influence nervous system function, mental function and emotions.

Hypnotherapy

What is it? A therapist hypnotises the patient. When totally relaxed, the patient can be relieved of stress, allergies or even physical addictions such as smoking.

Effect? It is based on positive thinking – that the power of a patient's own mind can bring about their healing.

Examples of alternative or complementary medicine

Homeopathy

What is it? Patients take a medicine (a plant, animal or mineral material soaked in alcohol) which causes similar symptoms to the illness they are suffering from.

Effect? The idea is that tiny doses of the medicine that causes similar symptoms will cure the patient by stimulating his or her natural defences. Studies have shown homeopathy to be effective in treating hay fever, insomnia, depression and eczema.

Key Words

positive health   alternative medicine

Acupuncture

What is it? Fine needles are placed at key points around the body. The places chosen are thought to be linked with particular needs or illnesses. Acupuncture has been a key part of traditional Chinese medicine for thousands of years.

Effect? The needles are said to release blocked energy and balance it properly. Acupuncture allows the energy to flow again; and it stimulates healing and relieves pain. It has been used as an anaesthetic during major surgery.

▼ **SOURCE C** *Acupuncture charts in an alternative therapy clinic*

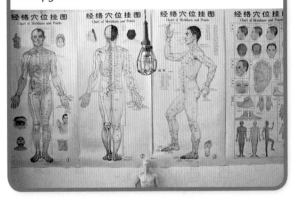

recent survey indicated that one in five people in Britain have consulted alternative healers and used alternative medicines. Today one in ten doctors is actively involved in the promotion of alternative medicine, and they sometimes offer 'complementary' medicine, which is when an alternative practice is used together with conventional medicine.

In recent years, there has been a greater emphasis placed on prevention rather than cure – this is sometimes known as 'positive health'. People are learning that regular exercise is very important for health; and that a good diet which avoids sugary, fatty foods can help prevent some of the twenty-first century's biggest killers, such as obesity and heart disease. There is also a lot of emphasis on making 'lifestyle changes' and publicising the dangers of tobacco and the misuse of alcohol and drugs.

There has also been an increase in screening, which focuses on checking people who seem to be healthy, aiming to find those who have the early signs of a serious illness like lung or breast cancer.

Work

1 Why do you think doctors and scientists are particularly worried about bacteria such as MRSA?
2 **a** What is meant by the term 'alternative medicine'?
   b Why has there been a rise in the popularity of alternative medicine in recent years?

Fact

One of the criticisms of alternative medicine is the lack of regulation. While mainstream medicine can only be practised by a doctor who has studied in medical school and been certified, alternative medicine can be prescribed by almost anyone. However, this is slowly changing as some alternative treatments such as osteopathy and chiropractic have professional regulations and licensing in the UK.

The impact of war and technology on surgery and health

11.1A

Throughout history, one of the key times when the latest medical techniques and the most up-to-date medical technology are needed is during wartime. If medical services are good, then more soldiers have a chance of survival; and the more soldiers there are available, the greater the country's chances of victory. Medicine usually develops at a greater rate during wartime than in peacetime. Governments pour a lot of money into developing ways of getting their injured soldiers back 'fighting fit' as soon as possible. Doctors and surgeons work very hard in wartime, often in battlefield situations, to develop their ideas in order to treat the injured. The huge numbers of wounded soldiers give doctors and surgeons more opportunities than are available in peacetime to test their ideas out.

Objectives

▶ **Examine** the links between the two world wars and medical progress.

▶ **Assess** the impact war and technology has had on surgery and health.

▶ **Explore** the latest technological breakthroughs since the Second World War, including radiation therapy and keyhole surgery.

The two world wars that took place during the twentieth century were huge conflicts that killed and wounded millions more people than in any wars before them. New and deadly weapons — high explosive shells, gas bombs, hand grenades and machine guns — were used on a massive scale for the first time, and inflicted terrible — often fatal — injuries. Over 10 million people were killed in the First World War (1914–18) and over 20 million in the Second World War (1939–45). These figures overlook the huge amount of people who were injured. Despite the great suffering caused by these two horrific wars, a number of improvements in surgery were made as a direct result.

Impact of the First World War on surgery

The diagram on these pages outlines the impact of the First World War on surgery and health. Advances made during and as a result of the Second World War are shown on pages 74 and 75.

Positives and negatives

As you can see from some of the examples on these pages, war can often bring about a great many medical developments and advances. But some historians argue that war can have a negative effect on medical progress too. For example, it could be argued that the First World War actually hindered the development of medicine because thousands of doctors were taken away from their normal work to treat casualties. Furthermore, lots of medical research was stopped during wartime so countries could concentrate everything on the war effort. Also, throughout history, warfare has disrupted towns and cities, sometimes destroying libraries and places of learning. Medical advances may have been delayed because these places were destroyed and manuscripts and research lost.

Work

1   In what ways can war have both a positive and a negative effect on the development of medicine?

2   Imagine you are an army surgeon in the First World War. Write a short letter home to your friends and family explaining how the latest scientific and technological developments have helped you in your work.

Shell shock

The mental strain of war could cause psychological damage known as shell shock. Some shell shocked soldiers had panic attacks; others shook all the time or were unable to speak or move. To begin with, the British army refused to believe that shell shock existed and many of the men were treated as cowards. However, by the end of the war, there were so many cases that shell shock was officially recognised. Today the condition is known as PTSD, or post-traumatic stress disorder.

Blood transfusions

Although blood transfusions had been tried for centuries, it wasn't until 1900 that scientists worked out how to do them successfully. Karl Landsteiner discovered blood groups, which helped doctors to work out that a transfusion only worked if the donor's blood type matched the receiver's. Even then it wasn't possible to store blood for long because it clotted so quickly. As a result, many people still died from loss of blood, so a solution to the problem of storing blood was needed. In 1914, Albert Hustin discovered that glucose and sodium citrate stopped blood from clotting on contact with air. Other advances meant that blood could be bottled, packed in ice, and taken to where it was needed by surgeons operating on soldiers.

X-rays

X-rays were discovered in 1895, and soon hospitals were using them to look for broken bones and disease. However, it was during the First World War that X-rays became really important. Mobile X-ray machines were used near battlefields to find out exactly where in the wounded soldier's body the bullets or pieces of shrapnel had lodged – without having to cut him wide open!

Plastic surgery

During the First World War, the hard work and dedication of Harold Gillies, a London-based army doctor, led to the development of what we now call plastic surgery. He set up a special unit to graft (transplant) skin and treat men suffering from severe facial wounds. He is commonly recognised as one of the first surgeons to consider a patient's appearance when treating wounds. Queen's Hospital in Kent opened in 1917 and by 1921 provided over 1000 beds for soldiers with severe facial wounds. Gillies and his colleagues treated over 5000 servicemen by 1921.

Infection

Battlefields are very dirty places and lethal wound infections such as gangrene were common. Through trial and error, surgeons worked out that the best way to prevent this was to cut away any infected flesh and soak the wound in salty (saline) solution. This wasn't ideal, but as a short-term answer in a battle situation, it saved many lives.

Broken bones

New techniques were developed during the First World War to repair broken bones. For example, the Army Leg Splint (or Keller-Blake Splint) was developed, which elevated and extended the broken leg 'in traction'. This helped the bones to knit together more securely. The splint is still in use today.

The impact of war and technology on surgery and health

The First World War sped up developments in surgery, health and medicine that probably would have happened anyway. For example, scientists had been working on blood transfusions for many years, but the amount of blood needed by soldiers in the war meant that scientists worked even harder to make blood transfusions a success. X-rays had been discovered in 1895, but it was during the First World War that X-ray technology became really important.

Impact of the Second World War on surgery and health

It was a similar situation in the Second World War. The millions of wounded soldiers meant that doctors, surgeons and scientists worked hard to develop new medicines and techniques – but they also tried to improve on some of the advances made in earlier years.

The National Health Service

When the Second World War broke out, the British government increased its involvement in medical care. After the war people started to think about how best to organise health care on a national basis. In 1942, a civil servant named William Beveridge proposed a free National Health Service for all – and just after the war finished, the NHS was born.

Blood transfusions

Advances in storing blood in the years after the First World War meant it could be kept fresh and useable for longer. This led to the British National Blood Transfusion Service opening in 1946. Large blood banks were developed in both the USA and Britain during the Second World War.

Heart surgery

Heart surgery progressed during the Second World War. American army surgeon Dwight Harken, stationed in London, cut into beating hearts and used his bare hands to remove bullets and bits of shrapnel. His findings helped heart surgery develop greatly after the war.

Impact of the Second World War on surgery and health in Britain

Plastic surgery

A doctor from New Zealand who trained and worked in Britain, Archibald McIndoe (a cousin of Harold Gillies), used new drugs such as penicillin to prevent infection when treating pilots with horrific facial injuries. His work on reconstructing damaged faces and hands was respected all over the world.

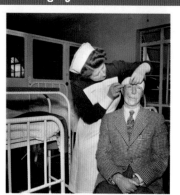

▲ SOURCE A *A soldier, wounded in the Second World War, after treatment by Archibald McIndoe*

Diet

Shortages of some foods during the war meant that the government encouraged people to grow their own food. This improved people's diets because the food they encouraged civilians to grow – fresh vegetables for example – was very healthy.

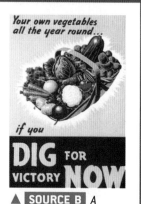

Your own vegetables all the year round…

if you

DIG FOR VICTORY NOW

▲ SOURCE B *A government poster issued during the Second World War*

Impact of technology on surgery

Major technological breakthroughs continued in the field of surgery after the world wars. Improved anaesthetics allowed patients to be unconscious for longer, so more complicated operations could be attempted; while better antiseptics increased the success rate of difficult operations because they cut down the chances of deadly infection. When transplant surgery became more common, new drugs helped to prevent a patient's body from 'rejecting' their new organs. Keyhole surgery, using small fibre-optic cameras linked to computers, meant surgeons could perform operations through very small cuts. Microsurgery allowed them to magnify the areas they were working on so they could re-join nerves and blood vessels – allowing feeling to be returned to damaged limbs.

Radiation therapy (also known as radiotherapy) has been used for the treatment of cancer and other diseases for over 100 years. However, the methods of treatment are developing all the time and it is estimated that about half of all cancer patients will receive some type of radiation therapy during the course of their treatment. Broadly speaking, radiation therapy involves the use of high-energy radiation to shrink tumors and kill cancer cells. The radiation may be delivered by a machine outside the body – or it may come from radioactive material placed inside the body near cancer cells. Sometimes a radioactive substance such as radioactive iodine is used, which travels in the blood to kill cancer cells.

Surgery using lasers (rather than a scalpel) has become increasingly popular since a laser was first used in an eye operation in 1987. Lasers are still commonly used in eye surgery, but are increasingly used to treat a variety of skin conditions, help clear blocked arteries, remove tumors and ulcers and control bleeding.

Why did the government try to improve the nation's health after 1900?

12.1A

Before the two world wars, the British fought a war in southern Africa called the Boer War (1899–1902). However, at the time around 40 per cent of the men who volunteered to fight were too unhealthy to be soldiers. In some big cities, 90 per cent of men weren't fit enough! This worried not only army leaders but also the British government too. But within five years of the end of the Boer War, the government had begun to introduce reforms aimed at getting Britain fitter and healthier – including free school meals for Britain's poorest children, school medical inspections, and a National Insurance Act which gave people the right to free medical treatment. So how exactly did the Boer War lead to free school meals? And what impact did the changes have on Britain's citizens?

Objectives

▶ **Explore** how and why public health was improved after 1900.

▶ **Outline** the Liberal social reforms of 1906 onwards in relation to poverty and housing in Britain.

▶ **Assess** the importance of Booth, Rowntree and the Boer War.

The Boer War

In 1899, a large-scale army recruitment campaign took place to find men to fight in the Boer War. But army chiefs were alarmed by the fact that 40 out of every 100 young men who volunteered were unfit to be soldiers – and the army didn't have particularly high entry standards either! The government was also shocked, so it set up a special committee to enquire into the 'Physical Deterioration of the People'. In 1904, the committee released its report. Among the many conclusions was the acknowledgement that many men were failing to get into the army because they led such unhealthy lives.

> ### Fact
> In the Boer War, the British and the Boers (descendants of Dutch settlers in Africa) competed for control of land in southern Africa.

The reports of Booth and Rowntree

Around the same time, several special investigations into the lives of the poor started to make headlines. For example, reports by Charles Booth, called *Life and Labour of the People in London*, found that around 30 per cent of Londoners were so poor that they didn't have enough

money to eat properly, despite having full-time jobs. He demonstrated that there was a link between poverty and a high death rate.

In York, Seebohm Rowntree's *Poverty: A Study of Town Life* (1901) found that 28 per cent of the population did not have the minimum amount of money to live on at some time of their life. This fuelled fears that the unhealthy state of Britain's workers could lead to the decline of the country as a great industrial power. Germany, for example, which had a good system of state welfare for workers, was beginning to produce as much coal, iron and steel as Britain.

These reports, and the Boer War itself, highlighted the fact that poverty and poor health had become one

▼ **SOURCE A** *An extract from Rowntree's* Poverty: A Study of Town Life *(1901):*

> These children presented a pathetic sight; all bore some mark of the hard conditions against which they were struggling. Puny and feeble bodies, dirty and often sadly insufficient clothing, sore eyes, in many cases acutely inflamed through continued want of attention, filthy heads, cases of hip disease, swollen glands – all these and other signs told a tale of neglect.

of the big issues of the time. They came at a time when more people were beginning to feel that one of the key responsibilities of any government was to look after people who can't look after themselves. Some politicians, including many from the Liberal Party (including Winston Churchill and David Lloyd George), believed that direct action from the government was the way to improve the public health, welfare and productivity of the nation. They were also worried about the popularity of the Labour Party, which had been founded in 1900, so they wanted measures that would appeal to working people and stop them voting for Labour. In 1906, the Liberal Party won the general election, and set to work.

The Liberal social reforms

School meals

In 1906, the School Meals Act allowed local councils to provide school meals, with poor children getting a free meal. By 1914, over 158,000 children were having a free school meal every day. However, lack of food was only part of the problem.

THIS WEEK'S MENU

Monday: Tomato soup – Currant roly-poly pudding

Tuesday: Meat pudding – Rice pudding

Wednesday: Yorkshire pudding, gravy, peas – Rice pudding and sultanas

Thursday: Vegetable soup – Currant pastry or fruit tart

Friday: Stewed fish, parsley sauce, peas, mashed potato – Blancmange

▲ **B** *Bradford was the first city to offer free school meals. They were introduced at a time when research showed that a poor child was, on average, nine centimetres shorter than a rich one.*

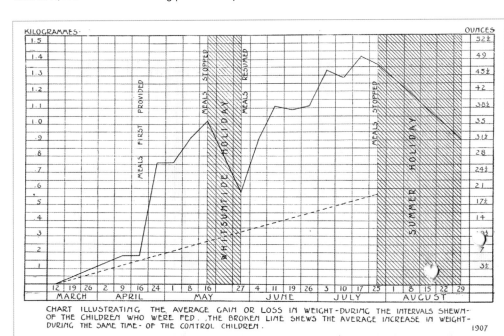

CHART ILLUSTRATING THE AVERAGE GAIN OR LOSS IN WEIGHT - DURING THE INTERVALS SHEWN - OF THE CHILDREN WHO WERE FED. THE BROKEN LINE SHEWS THE AVERAGE INCREASE IN WEIGHT - DURING THE SAME TIME - OF THE CONTROL CHILDREN. 1907

◄ **SOURCE C**
This graph from 1907 shows the impact of the free school meals; it charts the weight children gained (and lost) during part of the school year

Work

1 In what ways did the following affect the way the government felt about the health and welfare of British citizens: the Boer War; Charles Booth's report; Seebohm Rowntree's report; Germany.

2 Look at the menu in **B**.

   a Why were menus like this introduced in schools in the early 1900s?

   b Write down at least two reasons why many viewed this as a healthy menu.

c In what ways have modern governments today tried to improve the eating habits of young people at school?

3 Look at **Source C**.

   a What effect did providing meals have on the weight of the children?

   b What happened to the weight of the children during the holidays?

   c What is the dotted line – and why does the dotted line go up?

Why did the government try to improve the nation's health after 1900?

Children's health

In 1907, the government told all councils that they should have a school medical service. At first, doctors examined the children and then parents paid for treatment. When lots of parents failed to follow through with treatment – because they couldn't afford it – the government paid for school clinics to be set up with free treatment.

Other measures continued to help children. The Children and Young Person's Act of 1908, for example, made children into 'protected persons', which meant that parents were breaking the law if they neglected their children.

▼ **SOURCE D** *A school doctor consulting a mother during a medical examination of her young son, London 1911*

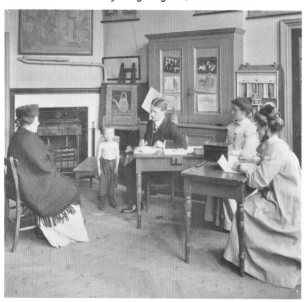

The school system was also seen as a way of improving children's health and well being. From 1907, special schools were set up to teach young women about the benefits of breastfeeding, hygiene and childcare.

Poverty and housing

After helping children, the government moved onto other sections of society. A National Insurance Act introduced unemployment benefit ('the dole'), free medical treatment and sickness pay. Old Age Pensions were introduced and Britain's first job centres were built.

▼ **SOURCE E** *Adapted excerpt from the Children and Young Person's Act, 1908. This was nicknamed 'The Children's Charter', and laid down in law many of the things that still protect children today:*

> Children are 'protected persons': parents can be prosecuted if they neglect or are cruel to them.
>
> Inspectors are to regularly visit any children who have been neglected in the past.
>
> All children's homes are to be regularly inspected.
>
> Youth courts and young offenders' homes are to be set up to keep young criminals away from older ones.
>
> Children under 14 are not allowed into pubs.
>
> Shopkeepers cannot sell cigarettes to anyone under 16.

Over the next 30 years, successive governments continued to take measures to improve the welfare of Britain's citizens. The building of overcrowded back-to-back housing was banned, for example, so fewer people would have to live in the crowded, filthy, disease-ridden slums. In 1918, local councils had to provide **health visitors**, clinics for pregnant women, and day nurseries. A year later, councils began to build new houses for poorer families and, by 1930, a huge slum clearance programme began, finally clearing away the breeding grounds of so much disease.

Impact of social reforms on public health

Gradually, during the twentieth century, infant mortality began to drop. A further boost to children's welfare was given in the 1940s with the introduction of the National Health Service (NHS). So, in today's world, health care begins before a baby is born: a pregnant woman will get free treatment and advice at antenatal clinics, and all hospital care and nursing are free. When the baby is born, it receives cheap milk, food and vitamins if required; then a free education, cheap (or free) school meals, dental treatment and eye care. And if a child has any need that requires a special school, for example if they are blind or deaf, this costs the parents nothing. In 2015, the infant mortality rate in the UK was 4.2 per 1000: meaning that for every one thousand babies born, fewer than five die before they are one year old.

Extension

Health issues are major news items. What topics related to health have been in this week's newspapers or TV news broadcasts?

Key Word

health visitor

▼ **SOURCE G** *A line graph showing the effect of a 1940 government campaign to get all children immunised against diphtheria; this disease causes a fever that makes sufferers short of breath, and it killed many children in the nineteenth century*

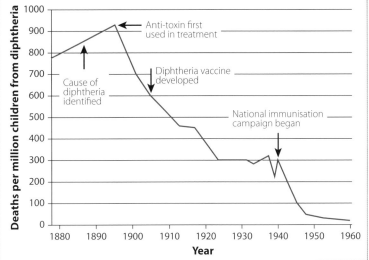

▼ **SOURCE F** *A bar graph showing infant mortality in Britain, 1840–2010*

Year	Deaths per child under one per 1000 live births
1840	150
1850	158
1860	152
1870	160
1880	140
1890	152
1900	163
1910	110
1920	80
1930	60
1940	55
1950	25
1960	20
1970	17
1980	15
1990	6
2000	5
2010	4

Work

1 Apart from the introduction of school meals, how else were children helped in the early 1900s?

2 Study **Source F**. In pairs or in groups, discuss why the infant mortality rate dropped between 1900 and 1945. You may want to review what you learned about the impact of the two world wars (pages 72–75) to help you with the discussion.

3 Look at **Source G**. Why do you think a national immunisation campaign for diphtheria was started in 1940?

Practice Question

Explain the significance of the Liberal social reforms for the prevention of disease. **8 marks**

Study Tip

Refer to different groups of people at the time and how the reforms relate to the NHS.

Into the twenty-first century

There is almost no-one in Britain who isn't helped at some time or another by the **welfare state**. This is the name of the system by which the government aims to help those in need, mainly the old, the sick, the unemployed and children. You and your family will almost certainly have been helped out by this system at one time or another. Sometimes also known as 'social security', the welfare state aims to ensure that nobody goes without food, shelter, clothing, medical care, education or any other basic need simply because they can't afford it. How did Britain develop into a welfare state in the twentieth century? What are the issues for public health in the twenty-first century?

Objectives

▶ **Examine** the impact of the two world wars on public health.

▶ **Explore** the concept of the welfare state and the development of the NHS.

▶ **Evaluate** the impact of the NHS.

▶ **Explore** the costs, choices and issues relating to healthcare in the twenty-first century.

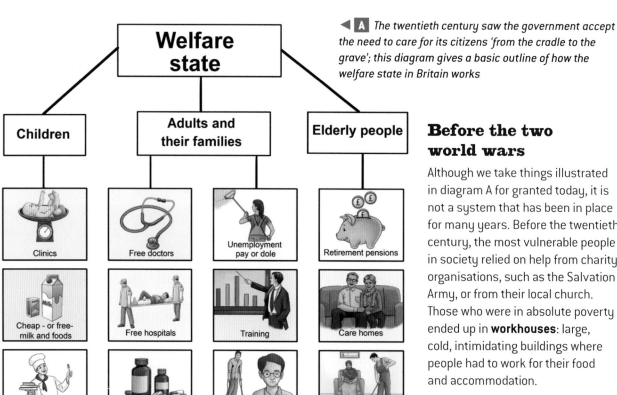

A The twentieth century saw the government accept the need to care for its citizens 'from the cradle to the grave'; this diagram gives a basic outline of how the welfare state in Britain works

Welfare state

Children

Clinics

Cheap - or free-milk and foods

Cheap - or free - school dinners

Education

Free dental care and spectacles

Adults and their families

Free doctors

Free hospitals

Cheap medicines

Family allowances

Sick pay

Unemployment pay or dole

Training

Pensions for those unable to work

Money for those on no income or only very small incomes

Maternity grants

Elderly people

Retirement pensions

Care homes

Home help

Meals at home

Financial help with funeral costs

Before the two world wars

Although we take things illustrated in diagram A for granted today, it is not a system that has been in place for many years. Before the twentieth century, the most vulnerable people in society relied on help from charity organisations, such as the Salvation Army, or from their local church. Those who were in absolute poverty ended up in **workhouses**: large, cold, intimidating buildings where people had to work for their food and accommodation.

From 1906, a few years after the Boer War ended, the government introduced some help for the most vulnerable sections of society: free school meals for poorer children, free school medical check-ups and treatment, small old-age pensions for the over 70s, and basic sick and 'dole' pay. But this was not on the same scale as what was introduced after the two world wars.

▼ **SOURCE B** *Speaking in 2006, Ivy Green from Nottingham remembers medical care in the 1930s:*

You paid National Insurance as soon as you got a job. We called it 'the stamp' and it worked like any insurance policy does today. You paid a set amount each week into a central fund and this entitled you to some basic sick pay and care from a 'panel doctor' if you were ill ... but because you only paid your stamp if you had a job, it meant you missed out on doctor's care when you lost your job. So when there was high unemployment in the 1930s, loads of people were unable to get any medical treatment because they hadn't been paying their stamp. You could pay for a doctor to visit you – six pence I think. It wasn't a lot of money but it still made you think twice about calling him. I'm sure lots of people mustn't have bothered to call a doctor because of the money.

Impact of the two world wars on public health

The death and destruction of the two world wars didn't just have an impact on people's lives – it had a major impact on attitudes too. It wasn't just the men fighting at the front that were dying: many people back in Britain suffered too, from shortages and bombing attacks. People felt that the sacrifices made at home and abroad should mean that the future should be a lot better for them. They felt that a better, fairer healthcare system should be part of this. And many middle-class people in the countryside had been genuinely shocked by the state of some of the dirty, under-nourished children who had been evacuated out of the cities during the Second World War. They felt that winning the wars should mean a better future for them too.

Beveridge Report

Towards the end of the Second World War, Sir William Beveridge wrote a report about the state of Britain. The Beveridge Report (1942) said that people all over the country had a right to be free of the 'five giants' that could ruin their lives:

- disease
- want (need)
- ignorance
- idleness
- squalor (very poor living conditions).

The report suggested ways to improve quality of life, and said that the government should 'take charge of social security from the cradle to the grave'. In a nation where people hoped that life would be better once the war was over, the report became a surprise bestseller, selling over 100,000 copies in its first month of publication.

Key Words

welfare state   workhouse

▼ **SOURCE C** *Sir William Beveridge (1879–1963)*

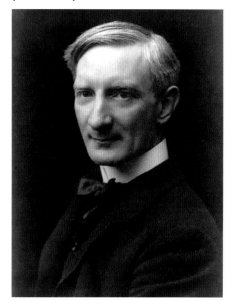

The Labour government

As the Second World War ended, an election was held to decide who would run the country after the war. The Labour Party promised to follow Beveridge's advice, while the Conservative Party, led by Winston Churchill, refused to make such a promise. The Labour Party won the election easily – and Winston Churchill, the man who had led Britain during the war, was out of power.

Work

1 In your own words, describe how the most vulnerable people in society were looked after before the Second World War.

2 a Explain what is meant by the term 'welfare state'.
  b What was the Beveridge Report?
  c In your own words, explain what you think was meant when the report said that the government should 'take charge of social security from the cradle to the grave'.

Into the twenty-first century

The welfare state

The new labour government, led by Clement Atlee, kept its promise: within the next few years, they put many of Beveridge's reforms into practice:

- The National Health Service (NHS) was set up in 1948 to provide health care for everyone. This made all medical treatment – doctors, hospitals, ambulances, dentists and opticians – free to all who wanted it.

- A weekly family allowance payment was introduced to help with childcare costs.

- The very poor received financial help or 'benefits'.

- The school leaving age was raised to 15 to give a greater chance of a decent education, and more free university places were created.

- The government's programme of 'slum clearance' continued as large areas of poor-quality housing were pulled down and new homes were built. Twelve new towns were created and by 1948, 280,000 council homes were being built each year.

Fact

The NHS scheme was originally opposed by doctors who didn't want to come under government control. Many felt that they would see a decline in their income because they could no longer charge what they wanted for their services. In a survey of around 45,500 doctors, nearly 41,000 didn't want a National Health Service! However, Aneurin Bevan, the Minister of Health, won them over by promising them a salary and allowing them to treat private patients as well.

Development of the NHS

Aneurin Bevan was the Minister of Health appointed by the government to introduce the NHS. And almost immediately, the NHS made an enormous impact. Up until 1948, around eight million people had never seen a doctor because they couldn't afford to. Now everyone could get free medical treatment and medicines.

It seems that Bevan's words hit home with health care providers – women's needs became a priority and they are now four times more likely to consult a doctor

▼ **SOURCE D** *From a speech by Aneurin Bevan in 1946:*

A person ought not to be stopped from seeking medical assistance by the anxiety of doctors' bills ... medical treatment should be made available to treat rich and poor alike in accordance with medical need and no other criteria. Worry about money in a time of sickness is a serious hindrance to recovery apart from its unnecessary cruelty. Records show that it is the mother in the average family who suffers most from the absence of a full health service. In trying to balance her budget she puts her own needs last.

▼ **SOURCE E** *From an interview with Frederick Rebman, speaking in 2004, remembering the introduction of the NHS:*

We were sorry to see Churchill voted out – he was our war leader, but he never promised to give the new ideas a go. The Labour Party did you see, and they publicised this in all the papers ... servicemen like me expected so much after the war, perhaps Utopia, and the welfare state seemed to be a good start. I didn't mind paying a bit more of my salary to know that a doctor or a dentist was there if I needed them. I felt it was worth it, that the government cared about us a bit more I suppose. I think there was a bit of a rush when the NHS first started. There were stories of people going and getting whole new sets of teeth, new glasses, even wigs. Perhaps they'd have struggled on before with their short-sightedness or their painful teeth, but now they didn't have to.

than men. Life expectancy for women has risen from 66 to 83 since 1948, and for men the figure has risen from 64 to 79. However, even in these modern times, your life expectancy can be affected by your wealth and living conditions. For example, in 2014, life expectancy for newborn baby boys was highest in the wealthy London areas of Kensington and Chelsea (83.3 years) and lowest in Blackpool (74.7 years), where there is far less wealth.

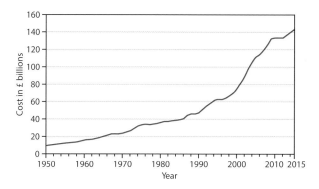

Costs of the welfare state

Of course, this all cost money. All workers had to pay for the NHS service through taxation, and over the years, the cost of welfare state services like the NHS rocketed. In fact, the NHS did not stay totally free for long. Working people today have to pay for doctors' prescriptions and dental treatment, for example, but the NHS ensures that no one is deprived of services such as family planning, physiotherapy, child care, cancer screening, asthma clinics and minor surgery simply because they can't afford it.

Healthcare in the twenty-first century

The NHS is rarely out of the news, mainly due to the fact that it has problems: waiting lists seem to be getting longer and doctors and nurses are overworked. There is rarely a month that goes by without some big media scandal about 'dirty wards', 'crumbling hospitals' or 'nurses doing long hours', or a news headline such as 'Doctors strike in UK-wide protest over pensions'. The main problem, of course, is money. Modern drugs are very expensive and modern medicine means that people are living longer – so there are more elderly people than ever before, and older people tend to use the services of the NHS more than younger people. The NHS has always been, and should continue to be, a really hot topic in British society.

The quest to improve medical treatments and public health continues today. Healthy eating campaigns and new laws try to protect Britain's citizens and prevent them from needing expensive medical care in the future. Tobacco advertising, for example, was banned in 2005 and in 2007 a smoking ban made it illegal to smoke in all enclosed public places. In 2015, drivers in England were banned from smoking in cars while carrying children as passengers.

Initiatives such as checking for the early signs of cancer, understanding how to spot (and deal with) a potential stroke victim, and trying to encourage people to eat five portions of fruit and vegetables a day are all aimed at making Britain healthier. In 2016, the British government unveiled plans to introduce a 'sugar tax', adding an additional cost to the price of high-sugar drinks, particularly fizzy drinks.

Technological breakthroughs and developments will also continue to improve the health and wellbeing of people. 'Digital therapy', for example, is designed for patients who need at-home care or who can't travel to a doctor's surgery or hospital. It is hoped that, in the future, mobile technology, combined with artificial intelligence (AI), will provide patients with a daily to-do list and a tracker for diet and exercise, based on results provided from patient scans.

Work

1 How did Beveridge and the Labour government win doctors over to accept the NHS?

2 Read **Source D**.
   a Who was Aneurin Bevan?
   b What point does he make about women in his speech?

3 Read **Source E**.
   a According to the source, why did the Labour Party win the election in 1945?
   b Why do you think people rushed out to get 'whole new sets of teeth, new glasses, even wigs' when the NHS first started?

4 Why do you think the NHS is still such a controversial topic today?

Practice Question

Have governments been the main factor in the development of public health?

16 marks

SPaG: 4 marks

Study Tip

Write about two more factors, for example, the role of individuals and religion. Refer to earlier periods in your answer.

How to... analyse significance

In your exam, you will have to deal with a question about analysing the significance of something, such as an event, an issue or a person.

Practice Question

Explain the significance of the work of William Harvey.   **8 marks**

Study Tip

Judging the *significance* of a person (such as Harvey) is about looking at the impact that he or she had *at the time*, how his or her work affected people *in the long term*, and whether his or her work is still relevant *today*.

Over to you

When we say an event, idea or person is *significant*, we mean more than just that it is important. Judging the significance of an event, idea or person is about looking at the impact that it had *at the time* and how it affected people, and whether it had long-lasting effects or caused important change. You should also consider whether the event, idea or person is still *relevant* to the present day. Now, work through the following questions.

1   Start by planning out your response: what do you know about the work of William Harvey? Make notes about what Harvey did at the time.

2   Consider Harvey's impact at the time of his discovery. Write about how people thought or did things before Harvey completed his work, and why Harvey's work was a change compared with what went before.

3   After you have written about Harvey's impact at the time, move on to consider how his work might have an impact in the long term.

4   Lastly, does Harvey's work directly affect our world today? Remember that the significance of an event, idea or person can *change* over time, so sometimes a lot of time will need to pass before it is recognised as being significant. Something might not be seen as particularly important *at the time*, but years later, when more is known, they can be identified as having had a key impact. Equally, something that was significant at the time may lose its significance as a result of later developments, and no longer influence our thinking or world *today*. So, considering all these points, what do *you* think is Harvey's significance?

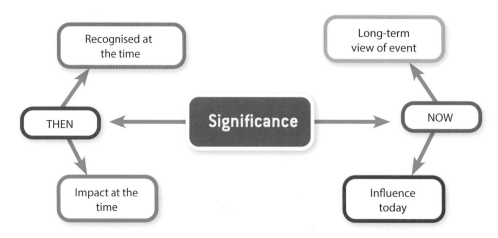

5 Read the following response. Can you identify where the answer explains about recognition of Harvey's work at the time, his immediate impact as well as his long-term impact, and his relevance today?

Harvey's discovery was recognised at the time as a great challenge to Galen's ancient ideas. There were arguments between those who supported Galen and those who supported Harvey's new theory. Harvey's discovery was not immediately useful for treatments, and further scientific discovery was needed. Eventually, however, in his lifetime the theory was accepted as correct.

At the time, Harvey's ideas about the circulation of blood weren't really seen as useful because they didn't help cure people.

But, the ideas prompted other scientists to carry out experiments.

Harvey experimented and used a scientific approach. Before Harvey, in the Middle Ages doctors studied Galen without questioning his ideas. In the Renaissance, Vesalius believed in showing people how the body worked through dissection.

In the seventeenth century, Harvey was increasing medical knowledge and learning through scientific experimentation. However, doctors still couldn't replace blood or do blood transfusions until 1901 when they knew more about blood groups. Still, understanding the circulation of the blood was a vital stage in the development of surgery and the diagnosis of illness. There are lots of modern medical techniques that could not work unless we understood about the circulation of the blood, such as blood tests and heart transplants.

6 Now try to answer the Practice Question on page 92 yourself!

How to... analyse sources

In your exam, you will have to deal with a question about analysing the usefulness of a source to a historian studying a particular area of history. You will be asked a question that directly relates to a source.

▼ **SOURCE A** *Drawn in 1802 by a British cartoonist, this picture is generally thought to show Edward Jenner giving his patients 'the new inoculation' at St Pancras Hospital in London. However, historians have suggested that the doctor is actually William Woodville, who ran the hospital. He was in dispute with Jenner after some of his patients died from smallpox when he used Jenner's technique.*

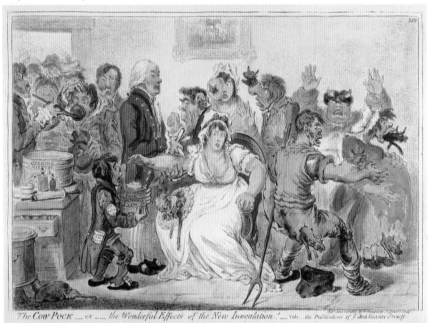

The Cow-Pock — or — the Wonderful Effects of the New Inoculation! — vide. the Publications of ŷ Anti Vaccine Society.

Practice Question

Study **Source A**. How useful is **Source A** to a historian studying vaccination?

8 marks

[Taken from AQA 2016 Paper 2 specimen material]

Study Tip

The provenance (for example, the place and date of publication, the type of source, and the title) can help you assess the usefulness of a source. What do you know about the topic that you can link with the information from the provenance?

Study Tip

The content of the source is the image itself. Begin by describing what you can see. What do you know about the history of vaccination that you can connect with what you see in the image?

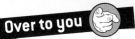

The usefulness of a source is what it could tell you about the history of the time. A source might be useful because it reveals something new, why events turned out the way they did or why people acted or thought in a particular way at that time. This question suggests that the source has a use for historians studying vaccination: remember this as you work through the following questions.

1 Start by analysing the content of **Source A**. Describe what you see. What is the cartoonist trying to say about vaccination? And what does it tell us about the topic that makes it useful or not? The content of the source should be checked against your own knowledge of the topic.

2 You should also consider the provenance of **Source A**:

   a What does it tell you about how useful, or not, the source might be? Provenance could mean who produced the source, why it was produced, who it was produced for, where and when it was produced. Remember that to asses the usefulness of a source, the provenance of a source is just as important as the content.

   b What was the context of the time in which the source was created? This source dates from 1802, which was only a few years after Jenner's discovery about cowpox. The provenance suggests that this is not Jenner but another doctor using Jenner's method. Perhaps you could argue that this source is useful because it gives historians the evidence that Jenner's method is popular because someone else is using it.

3 Recall the actual question: it asks about a historian studying vaccination. In **Source A**, the patients are growing small cows from different parts of their body, which suggests that the cartoonist does not approve of vaccination. Why might this be? It is helpful if you try to use the provenance and the content together. The provenance said that some patients had died from smallpox when using Jenner's technique. It might seem that vaccination did not work. Do you remember that people used inoculation before vaccination? Perhaps the cartoonist thinks that inoculation is safer.

4 What are the strengths and weaknesses of the following answer?

> The source is useful because it comes from near the time when Jenner made his discovery in 1798 about vaccination. So the source will show what people were thinking at the time about vaccination. The picture shows people with cows growing out of them and this suggests that the cartoonist didn't understand how vaccination worked and thought there would be bizarre side effects — or it just wouldn't work. The cartoonist seems to be poking fun at vaccination. The provenance suggests that people had come across severe side effects like death! The source is useful because it shows the historian that people did not accept vaccination immediately. I know that people were inoculated with weak smallpox to give immunity. Doctors made a lot of money from this. Perhaps the cartoonist prefers those doctors and their methods. At the time, Jenner could not explain why his method worked so people were reluctant to accept it. If doctors used Jenner's method incorrectly or with dirty instruments they could infect people with smallpox.

5 Now try to answer the Practice Question on page 92 yourself!

How to... compare similarities

In your exam, you will have to deal with a question about analysing the similarities of two things, such as two events or developments.

Practice Question

Explain two ways in which the Black Death in the Middle Ages and the cholera epidemics in the nineteenth century were similar.

8 marks

Study Tip

Write something about both events, and explain the similarities between their causes, development and consequences.

Over to you

This style of question asks you to explain the similarities between two topics or aspects of the history you have studied. You are looking for similarities between the two events: remember this as you work through the following questions.

1   Start by planning out your response: what are the similarities between the Black Death and cholera epidemics? Make a list or mind-map to help you analyse the similarities. For example, when comparing events, consider:

   a   causes: why did the event happen?

   b   development: how did the event develop?

   c   consequences: events will have results.

2   Try to organise your response in three sections, covering causes, development and consequences. Remember that you will need to show how well you have understood both events by explaining the similarities that you can find.

3   Read the following response. Can you identify where the answer explains about similarities in terms of causes, development and consequences?

> Cholera came to England in 1831. It killed lots of people who lived in low-quality housing and who often had a water supply that was contaminated with sewage. A shared water supply was an easy way for the disease to spread. The Black Death also had an easy way to spread. The Black Death was two sorts of plague, one pneumonic, the other bubonic, so it could be spread by a flea's bite but also by droplets in the

breath of someone who was infected. Because both diseases spread so easily, many thousands of people died from both diseases. Both the Black Death and cholera led to changes in the lives of those people who survived it. Cholera drew attention to the dirty living conditions in towns and cities. This influenced the work of people like Chadwick and Farr who believed that cleanliness would reduce disease. The disease, and the terrible living conditions in which it thrived, led to new laws such as the Public Health Acts in 1848 and 1875. So cholera contributed to better sanitation through legislation. The Black Death killed so many people in Medieval times that those who survived received better wages in the decades after the Black Death. This was because England was agricultural and the landowners needed the hard work of the ordinary people to bring in harvests and tend the land. So the epidemics are similar because they had a big impact on those who survived them.

4   As you can read, this answer explains the similarities between both events for the way they developed and their consequences. Can you write a paragraph that explains the similarities between both events for a similar aspect connected with what caused each epidemic?

5   Now try to answer the Practice Question on page 92 yourself!

How to... evaluate main factors

In your exam, you will have to deal with a question that asks you to evaluate factors.

Over to you

Different factors have affected this Health and the People thematic study over a long period of time. Those factors are war, superstition and religion, chance, government, communication, science and technology and the role of the individual in encouraging or inhibiting change. Frequently, factors worked together to bring about particular developments at particular times. It is important that you show an understanding of this, and how they were related to each other and their impact upon society. Remember this as you work through the following questions.

1   Start by writing about the factor that has been named in the question: in this case, it is about the role that science and technology played in developing the treatment of disease in Britain. You will have come across examples where science and technology have appeared in your study of health and the people. Using these examples, write about how science and technology has had an influence. The factor you are addressing might sometimes have helped and sometimes hindered the treatment of disease. Try to give two or three examples from different times or places during your study.

2   Next, consider other factors that have influenced the treatment of disease, for example the role of different individuals or the way that war has made an impact. Choose two or three other factors from your study and explain, with examples, how those factors made an impact on the treatment of disease in Britain. Again, it is useful if you can find examples from across the wide range of your study that both helped and hindered the development.

3   Lastly, you will have to deal with the judgement in the question. The question picked out that science and technology was the main factor in developing the treatment of disease in Britain. You have to say whether or not you agree with this. Try to weigh up or assess the science and technology factor against other ones, and say which was more important. To back up your conclusion, you should also explain why, with supporting evidence.

4 Read the following extract from an essay answer. Can you identify: the given factor (science and technology) and another factor? The supporting points about each factor? An assessment or judgement about which is the main factor? What might be missing from this answer?

Science and technology have played an important role in developing the treatment of disease in Britain. As scientific understanding and methods developed, people understood the causes of diseases better, and how to treat them. In the Middle Ages, diseases like the Black Death were explained by people as a punishment from God. At this time, people did not know about germs — there were no microscopes powerful for them to see them. But, as technology improved and glass lenses became better in the late 1600s and early 1700s, scientists were able to see tiny organisms moving about in water droplets, food, and animal and human body parts. This led to detailed research on microbes and, consequently, scientists such as Pasteur and Koch made major breakthroughs in this area. Indeed, it was Pasteur who showed, through a series of experiments with a swan-necked flask, that germs cause disease. These ideas challenged older beliefs about miasma and spontaneous generation. Without Pasteur and Koch's scientific approach, and (for example) Lionel Beale's microscope work in relation to the cattle plague in June 1866, British doctors would not have been convinced about the relationship between microbes and disease. Joseph Lister, working in Britain in the 1860s, and his antiseptic approach can be linked to his recognition of Pasteur's Germ Theory.

The role of the individual has also been an important factor in the treatment of disease in Britain. Edward Jenner, for example, developed a vaccination for one of the most feared diseases of the eighteenth century — smallpox. Through repeated experiments, he concluded correctly that cowpox protected humans from smallpox, and published his findings (to much opposition) in 1798. Also, individuals such as Fleming, Florey and Chain have been important for their insight and dedication. For example, Howard Florey assembled a team, including Ernst Chain, to study the germ-killing powers of natural substances. They found Alexander Fleming's research on penicillin and had the background to approach things scientifically and grow, purify and test penicillin properly.

The two factors mentioned above relate to each other in several ways. For example, individuals such as Pasteur and Koch used the latest technology (such as state-of-the-art microscopes and precision equipment) whilst Florey and Chain embraced the latest developments in mass production. Other factors, such as government and war played a role too — the US government, for example, agreed to pay several huge chemical companies to make millions of gallons of penicillin, spurred on by a war that needed a steady supply of it to treat infected soldiers.

However, of the two main factors mentioned here, I think that science and technology is the most important factor. Without the scientific methods they apply to their work, and the technology (instruments, equipment, lenses, glass flasks, machinery etc) at their disposal, the individuals would not have made the advances they did. Although individuals like Jenner, Lister and Florey all show great determination and insight, they all work in a scientific way based upon measurable evidence. It is the work of science that persuades government to use its power and wealth to improve treatments.

5 Now try and answer the Practice Question on page 92 yourself!

Practice Questions for Paper 2: Britain: Health and the people: c1000 to the present day

The examination questions on the Health and the People exam will be varied but there will be a question on a source (AO3), a question on significance (AO1 and AO2), a similarity/difference question (AO1 and AO2), and an extended writing question using factors (AO1 and AO2). Below is a selection of these different kinds of questions for you to practise.

Answer **all four** questions. You are advised to spend 50 minutes on these four questions.

Source A

A cartoon from the satirical* magazine *Punch*, 1948. It shows the Minister for Health, Aneurin Bevan, giving doctors their NHS medicine. The title of the cartoon is 'It still tastes awful'.

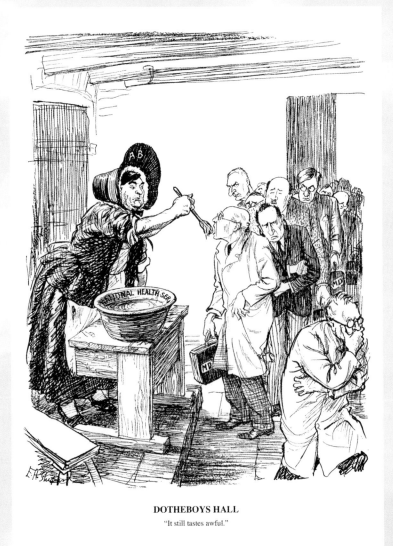

DOTHEBOYS HALL

"It still tastes awful."

*satirical = critical and humorous

1   Study **Source A**.

    How useful is **Source A** to a historian studying the creation of the NHS?

    Explain your answer using **Source A** and your contextual knowledge.   `8 marks`

2   Explain the significance of penicillin in the development of medicine.   `8 marks`

3   Explain two ways in which surgery in the Middle Ages and surgery at the time of John Hunter were similar.

    `8 marks`

4   Has the role of the individual been the main factor in understanding the causes of disease in Britain?

    Explain your answer with reference to the role of individuals and other factors.

    Use examples from your study of Health and the people.   `16 marks`
    `SPaG: 4 marks`

Glossary

alternative medicine term used to describe any other way of treating an illness or health condition that doesn't rely on mainstream, doctor-dispensed scientific medicine, or on proven evidence gathered using the scientific method; it contains a wide range of practices and therapies

anaesthetic substance that removes pain

anatomy science of understanding the structure and internal organs of the body

Ancient World period in Western history when Greek and Roman cultures and civilisations were at the heights of their power, from around 700BC to AD500

anti-contagionism belief that infection was caused when infectious matter interacted with the environment and created the disease, which affected weak individuals

antibiotic medications used to cure, and in some cases prevent, bacterial infections; they are not effective against viruses such as the common cold

antiseptic chemical applied to a wound to prevent the growth of disease-causing microbes; also applied to surgical instruments

aseptic state of being completely free of harmful microbes; sterilising to create a contamination-free environment

astrology study of the stars and planets

bacteria microorganisms that live in water, soil, plants and animals and that can cause diseases

bacteriologist someone who studies bacteria

barber-surgeon Medieval barber who practiced surgery and dentistry

bloodletting Medieval medical treatment of removing some blood from a patient by opening a vein or using leeches to suck it out

bubonic plague plague spread by the bite of a flea; buboes are lumps

Caliph ruler of the Islamic Empire

cauterisation using a heated iron to stop bleeding and seal a wound

cesspit pit for the disposal of liquid waste and sewage

cholera infectious and often fatal bacterial disease, usually contracted from infected water supplies and causing severe vomiting and diarrhoea

contagionism belief that infection was caused by contact with an infected person or germ

contagious spreadable

crusading order military monks who fought to gain control of the land of Christ's birth from Muslim rulers

diagnosis identification of a disease

dissection methodical cutting up of a body or plant in order to study its internal parts

DNA (deoxyribonucleic acid) molecules that genes are made from

emetic substance that makes a patient vomit

enema fluid injected into the bowel to clean it

epidemic spread of a disease to a large number of people

feudal system Medieval system of land holding and distribution in which the use of the land is paid for by performing services and work for the owner

Germ Theory theory that bacteria (germs) cause disease

gong farmer person who cleaned out privies or cesspits in Medieval times

health visitor qualified nurse or midwife with additional training and qualifications in public health; they assess the health needs of individuals, families and the wider community to promote good health and prevent illness

Human Genome Project international project to de-code and identify human genes

humours the theory of the four humours is based on the idea that everything was made of the four elements of fire, wind, earth and water; and that elements exist as different liquids in the body

inoculation using weakened but live germs of a disease in a healthy person to build up an immunity (resistance) against the stronger form of the same disease

keyhole surgery modern surgical technique in which operations are performed inside the body using cameras and instruments inserted through small incisions on the skin

laissez-faire French words meaning 'leave alone'; in the nineteenth century many people felt that this was what the government should do: not interfere, not force people to change, and allow things to take their own course

lavatorium communal washing area for monks

lay people ordinary people who were not monks or priests

leech blood-sucking worm-like insect

leprosy contagious disease that ate away parts of the victim's body, which would then become horribly deformed

miasma name given to what people thought was an 'infectious mist' given off by rotting animals, rubbish and human waste; many believed it caused illness and disease

microbe living organism that is too tiny to be seen without a microscope; includes bacteria, which can cause diseases

mould type of fungus that grows in thin threads, usually in warm, moist conditions

pandemic a disease that has spread across a large region - for example, multiple continents or worldwide

patron supporter or sponsor

pharmaceutical industry businesses that develop and produce drugs for use in medicine and health care

pilgrimage journey, of devotion or of moral significance, to visit a holy place

pneumonic plague plague spread by breathing in germs from the infected lungs of a bubonic plague victim

positive health focus on the prevention of illness and disease rather than the cure

privy toilet located in a small shed outside a house or building

public health health of the population as a whole

purgative laxative that makes you go to the toilet

purge physical removal of something or someone; normally carried out violently or abruptly

quack person pretending to have medical ability or fake cures; unqualified, often useless, doctor

quarantine confining or stopping people from going in or out of a place

Renaissance 'rebirth' or revival of European art and literature under the influence of classical ancient Greece and Roman models in the fourteenth to sixteenth centuries

screening checking for the presence of a disease

specificity theory that specific germs cause specific diseases

spontaneous generation theory that microbes appear as if by magic, and that germs are the result of disease

spore cell or small organism that can grow into a new organism in the correct conditions

trepanning drilling holes in the head

vaccination using the dead germs of a disease or one similar to it to build up an immunity (resistance) against the stronger form of the disease

vaccine substance that is injected into a person to protect against a particular disease

virus/viral infection infection caused by microbes which can be contagious; unlike bacterial infection, most viruses do cause diseases, and antibiotics cannot cure viral infections

welfare state system by which the government looks after the well-being of the nation, particularly those who cannot help themselves, such as the old, children, the sick and the unemployed

workhouse public institution in which the destitute of a parish received board and lodging in return for work

Index